MEDICINE THE DIRTY PROFESSION

A LIFE LONG STRUGGLE OF A MEDICAL DOCTOR

DR. NABIL BASANTI

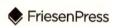

Suite 300 - 990 Fort St
Victoria, BC, V8V 3K2
Canada

www.friesenpress.com

Copyright © 2019 by Dr. Nabil Basanti
First Edition — 2019

All rights reserved.

No part of this publication may be reproduced in any form, or by any means, electronic or mechanical, including photocopying, recording, or any information browsing, storage, or retrieval system, without permission in writing from FriesenPress.

ISBN
978-1-5255-3491-1 (Hardcover)
978-1-5255-3492-8 (Paperback)
978-1-5255-3493-5 (eBook)

1. MEDICAL, ETHICS

Distributed to the trade by The Ingram Book Company

TABLE OF CONTENTS

PREFACE	V
INTRODUCTION	VII
CHAPTER 1	1
The Birth Of A Doctor	
CHAPTER 2	5
The Road To Medicine	
CHAPTER 3	17
The Reality of Practicing Medicine	
CHAPTER 4	41
Discovering Unprofessionalism	
CHAPTER 5	49
Discovering dirty Medicine in The USA	
CHAPTER 6	61
Terrible Experience of Medicine in the Arabian Gulf	
CHAPTER 7	73
Discovering real dirt in the American Medical System	
CHAPTER 8	81
Exploring Alternatives to Dirty Medicine	
CHAPTER 9	103
The Dirt in Medical Imaging	
CHAPTER 10	133
My Family and Medicine	
CHAPTER 11	155
Medical Radiation Technologists (MRT)	
CHAPTER 12	169
Doctors Identity and Health Systems	
ACKNOWLEDGEMENTS	179
ABOUT THE AUTHOR	181

PREFACE

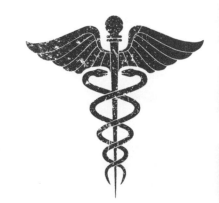

I have been trying to write this book for many years; yet, I was always discouraged by people around me. Everybody would tell me you have to be careful of mentioning any names of individuals or institutions, as they can cause problems for you. Others would say that there are people who have the ability to hurt you personally if you expose their dirty tactics. So, I kept delaying it, year after year, for the last five years.

I was in Europe when the catastrophe of the Charlie Hebdo massacre occurred, and it inspired me to write about my experiences—the dirt I have faced and endured within the medical profession. After witnessing millions of people worldwide holding up their pens and signs of "*Je suis Charlie*" expressing the freedom of speech that all people should experience, I decided to write my book.

INTRODUCTION

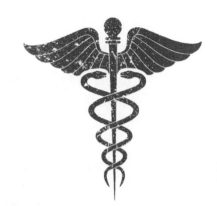

This is a book that exposes incidents and episodes from the heroic medical practice I was involved in, to the dirty, greedy medical practice in the modern world that I was part of as a medical radiation technologist, owner of a couple of private imaging clinics and an advisor for mending broken health systems. It is written:

> For all those **good honest doctors** to ascertain how some of their colleagues are practicing.
>
> For all the **bad doctors** to awaken their conscious, abort their dirty practices and focus on their mission to help the sick.
>
> For all *foreign-trained doctors* who have the dream of moving to the so-called civilized world, to expect the unexpected.

For all the ***sick people*** to be careful in doing their due diligence in researching their illness and discussing it with their doctor. The internet is not a good source of research, the best references are medical books in the medical libraries. Always get a second opinion for major illness and never believe what any doctor would say, you never know what motives they have.

For the ***healthy people*** as a means of entertainment, reading with equipped knowledge of what the current medical profession has to offer, so when the time comes and they are sick, they will be predetermined to be careful and know how to handle their illnesses.

For the ***students who intend to study medicine,*** so they will not be disappointed.

For the ***practicing and future medical radiation technologists*** to be aware of how their identity is viewed in the health system.

I hope this book will serve the non-prejudiced purpose for which it is written and with the grace of the almighty Lord, God our creator and savior, will bring out the good in people.

CHAPTER 1

The Birth Of A Doctor

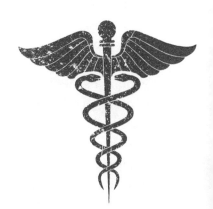

On a late July afternoon of 1954, in a North African country falling close to the equator and the Sahara Dessert, the temperature was about 40°C, and a twenty-year-old woman gave birth to a son. This was her second child from a husband who was an architect working with the Egyptian army to rebuild the country infrastructure after independence from the British monarchy.

In the early fifties, child delivery was a matter of life and death in the under-developed world. There were no equipped hospitals with maternity suites to accommodate child delivery. Deliveries were conducted by midwives. The midwife in this particular birth drove a very old black car and upon arriving at the pregnant woman's house guided the mother through a successful vaginal delivery, and a seven pound baby boy was born. Of course, midwives were experts in delivering babies especially during that time and place as female circumcision was the norm on that side of the world. Yet, in spite of the midwife's expertise, the mother developed post-partum hemorrhage and on the midwife's recall, she examined the mom and discovered that she had left behind a small portion of the placenta which was then removed. The mother was lucky to survive and did so without the need of a blood transfusion or further treatment.

The mother was from a well-off family and had a fair share of education in a Catholic missionary school. In the villages, on the other hand, especially in the southern parts of the country, delivering a child was a huge risk, yet astonishingly, many make it, and both the child and mother survive. The unlucky families lose either the child or the mom. In the village, when a pregnant woman feels her water break, she stops working in the fields and tries to walk to a shady area if the delivery is during the day and or a moon lighted area if the delivery is at night.

The mother in the villages, selects a low tree branch where she can squat, bending her knees and still able to reach the tree branch. She holds the branch with both her hands and keeps pushing to deliver her baby. The mom usually places a piece of cloth or rug under herself so she can deliver her baby without him getting covered in the dirt of the grass, soil, or sand. When the baby is delivered, his mom lays the baby on her side and maneuvers the placenta out by pulling on the umbilical cord and, if needed, reaches for the branch with the other hand, pushing until the placenta is delivered. Then she ties the cord in a knot and places the umbilical cord on a big smooth rock and hits it with a smaller sharp-edged stone several times till it is cut off. The mom picks up the baby stimulating it to have the first breath, wiping the nose and mouth of any mucus or dirt so the baby can breathe. When the placenta is delivered, the mom throws it away and picks up her baby, cuddles him, gives him a breast to feed and then lies down to rest. When she is rested she ties the baby on her back and walks back to the village to her family.

The Birth Of A Doctor

What a contrast of events in the 1950's—the city-boy grows up and develops to be a doctor, while the village-boy's future was undetermined and faced with infectious diseases, malnutrition and uncertainty for survival. But life goes on anywhere and each individual faces a destiny that is beyond his/her control.

When the young mom was in her early twenties with two sons aged two years and one year, the family sadly discovered that her husband, the architect, was involved in heavy gambling with the Egyptian soldiers and also involved in drug trafficking. The husband's father sent him a letter that accidentally reached the young boys' grandad stating that the Government in Egypt was cracking down on all drug dealers and that he might be on the watchlist so for his safety should avoid returning back there.

This letter was a key resource for applying for divorce to the patriarch of the Coptic Church, the late Kyrollas VI, who wisely issued a divorce decree after collecting the facts about the children's father from drug dealings to gambling and neglect of the wife and children. A decree was issued and the mom got custody of the children and returned to live in her dad's house. The two sons lived with their mom, grandparents, and three uncles. The children were loved and taken care of. They were given the best education and were brought up with very strong Coptic Orthodox Christian doctrines.

The young boy was always interested in treating medical problems. Any time there was need for eye drops to any family member, the boy was encouraged to come and deliver the drops. Any minor wound that came across the family, the boy was called to clean the wounds, apply cleansers, and place dressings. The young boy enjoyed it and all members of the family knowing his interest hoped that one day he would be a doctor.

CHAPTER 2

The Road To Medicine

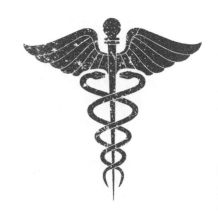

When it was time for school, my older brother and I were enrolled in a private missionary primary and secondary Catholic school named for Father Comboni, a catholic preacher, who died in one of the provinces while he was preaching. **Comboni College** was staffed mainly by Italian priests for it was the only legal way church missionaries could have visas as teachers in a school in a Muslim country. Catholic nuns hosted both primary and secondary schools for girls, having the same visa arrangement as school teachers. The schools were filled with multicultural values since all the business people in that country were Italians, Greeks, Armenians, Jews, Ethiopians, Lebanese, English, French, Germans, Americans and Syrians. The kids of these cultures were enrolled in Comboni College since it was considered a prestigious place of education where only the rich can afford to send their kids. For the same reason, some of the rich high-class Muslim local kids also enrolled due to the business relationship of their families with these cultures.

English was the lingua franca at Comboni College and all subjects were taught in English; thus, we depended on hard work and our priest teachers to succeed. In fact, Arabic was the only subject that was difficult and needed a tutor from school to help. My grandfather was well versed in the English language and he was our English teacher. For Arabic, we had help from another family member well acquainted with the language, and for the upper classes, an Arabic teacher used to come to our house. My brother was two years ahead of me; he and I had a math teacher since all our courses were in English. My uncles, unfortunately, were not that strong in English. Math was a challenge for my uncles since they had all their education in Arabic, even in university, when they were enrolled in finance and law. In the last year of secondary school, we were kind of on our own for calculus and algebra complicated the math prerequisite and we relied on the teaching priests at school.

Elementary school was far from our house, so we used to take the school bus. The four years of elementary were normal with not much excitement. The primary school was close to our house in the centre of the capital. My uncle used to drive us for the first few years and in the later years we would walk with friends. I was very competitive in primary school and used to be the first of my class; occasionally there was Brian, the English boy who used to compete with me for top of the class. Neil was another Indian boy who competed with both of us, so if I was not the first of my class, one of my friends would be, and we three shared the top three rankings in the primary years. The school had very organized gymnastic programs in which we exercise regularly to prepare for the end of the year gymnastic show (called Display) that hosted all students.

My grandparents were very protective, and, as a result, we were only allowed to have friends to come to *our* house in the school holidays during the summer. Occasionally, we might go to the Coptic club where we played basketball and hung out with friends from the same neighbourhood community. At that time television was a rarity and only in black and white. Sometimes we were allowed to go watch a movie at our neighbour's place where they had a television. Families were very friendly, they visit each other, and all the boys and girls mingled with each other with peace and love. All families knew each other and knew where their kids were and with whom they were mingling. Advice and protection surrounded the community with closeness to the Church where priests used to nourish the community with prayer and faith.

On entering the secondary school, the first year was the decisive year where students would pick up their specialization either in the scientific section or the commercial section. Students were streamed depending on their grades: the students with high grades were selected for science; those with average or low grades were selected for commerce. My brother was already in the scientific section, but I got mixed with a group of other teenage kids and started making fun of the teachers and priests and stayed at the back row of the class. One of the funny kids' stuff I recall was that when the teacher asks if we understood, we were six kids that all said 'yes'. Each of us would say yes, so that there were six yeses in a row. We were appropriately labelled the "yes gang".

After the first three months reports came out; my marks were very low: I nearly flunked all eight subjects. I remember I scored 10 in English Literature. My brother together with the headmaster talked to me and told me that I would fail the grade if I continued this way and that I had to straighten out and concentrate on my studies or else I might end up repeating the grade. The headmaster broke up the "yes gang" and brought me to the first row of the class in front of the teacher`s desk. My family got notice of my situation; they were very supportive and helped me to study more and try to get better grades. The second semester I got passing grades, the third semester, higher grades and in the fourth, I achieved superior grades high enough to pass the grade required to enroll in science classes. The priest headmaster told my brother that this student had showed such a super effort to reach the end of the grade with passing results from severely flunking in the first semester, he earned the right to be accepted in the science section of the school. That was a turning point in my road in education; I was rewarded by being accepted into the scientific section enabling me to try to fulfil my dream of becoming a physician.

The last three years of secondary school was spent in science with the pleasure of dissections in biology and strengths in physics and chemistry with a harmonized discovery of just how much living things and environment are interconnected. The priest who taught us biology, Fr. Denicolo, had a very good relationship with me and he allowed me to explore lots of demonstrations in the lab and explained things thoroughly with me grasping nearly all the curriculum in biology and botany. The priest, who taught physics, Fr. Charles, was also kind and helpful and I was allowed to work a great deal in the physics laboratory where lots of physical phenomena were executed practically. The chemistry priest also helped enormously by allowing me to work in the chemistry lab on many things from conducting simple chemical experiments to discovering unknown elements. I was always participating in the school's science open house, when it was conducted, participating in all scientific modalities.

There was a university teacher who used to teach us math and calculus. A friend of mine who used to sit next to me in class was a math genius and he helped me whenever I needed to solve complicated problems. As a whole, all tutors liked me for I showed a high interest in learning the sciences and I showed very high grades all through. We were a class of 45 students. The most competitive were myself and Mustafa, the math genius, and Wagdi who seemed to always get higher than both of us. That last year secondary school group was an amazing group. We were very noisy and active, the headmaster had to move our class next to his office in a science lab class to try and control us, and we used to knock on the wall to get his attention when we needed to give him hard time. In the school history, our class was the only student group where the last student in the group had an average of 55. Nobody had any failures and amazingly all the group ended in being admitted to different universities all over the world.

At that time, there was only one university in the country. It was affiliated with Oxford University in England. All the rules and regulations for enrolling in the university were dictated by the English affiliation to keep the international level of grades competitive. For admission to Medical school, the student must qualify for enrolling in an advanced 'A - level' which is the first year of university in general science where at the year's end an additional competition will take place and the highest scoring student will be qualified to enroll in Medicine if they elected it as their career choice.

Knowing the system, admission was possible by aggregating scores from Science subjects, from more than one secondary school certificate. I convinced some of my friends to sit for the Oxford general certificate where the exams come from Oxford University in England. We sat for the Sciences and Math subjects so it could be a buffer in admission in case it was needed when we sat for the local government secondary school certification which was conducted by the government ministry of education.

I remember the timing of the government secondary school certificate was pushed to conflict with the timing of Oxford general certificate because the government wanted to deter students studying in the private Christian school from using the privilege of aggregating any subjects towards enrolling in the University. All schools in the country had their curriculum in Arabic and the students were unable to sit for the English Oxford examinations. To serve their students, the college made an agreement with Oxford University to allow exams to be conducted in the afternoon instead of the mornings to allow students who are interested to sit for the exams. Oxford University allowed the Oxford exams to be run in the afternoons, while the government secondary school certificate exams were conducted in the mornings. So, we ended up taking exams from the secondary school certificate in the morning while returning in the afternoon for the Oxford exams.

On the first day of the government secondary school exams, astonishingly, I discovered that one of my close friends, Nigel, sat doing nothing in the morning government secondary school certificate, and wanted to leave after few minutes of distributing the exam questions. He was not allowed to leave till the last 15 minutes of the three hour exam. At that time, there were five exam questions and they were all essay type. Multiple choice questions did not exist in the English system. When we finished, I asked him, and he told me that he had the exam questions the night before at his house and it is unfair to write the exam knowing that other students and friends didn't have the same questions before. Strangely enough, the student friends whom I convinced to sit for the Oxford exam had access to the exams and never came around to share with me. We found out that somebody had his galabia, the traditional dress in the country, pushed in the printing press and got all the exam questions printed on his dress shirt. They were sold to some parents, but I never had access to any of them.

We continued to take exams mornings and evenings for seven days. After few days, the ministry of education announced cancelling all the exams from the government secondary schools all around the country and rescheduled the exams to a postponed date. Those who registered for the Oxford exams continued the evening cession examination and we had to again prepare for retaking the government high secondary school exams.

Thirteen thousand students sat for the secondary school certificate exams in the scientific section. For the 'A Level' General Science entry requirements, only 750 top students would be selected. I was ranked 500 for I had the second highest grade in the country for biology as I was told at a later date.

I was admitted in the General Science 'A-Level' department of the University. That was a very prestigious challenging incidence for it was the first step towards the road to medical school. I had to compete with the other 750 students to be on the top 180 since admission to medical school accepts the highest 180 students. Working very hard and studying with concentration, I scored 2 As and a B+ in zoology, botany and chemistry, that ranked me as the 85th student in the required 180 selection and was admitted to the Faculty of Medicine at the University. Few friends from my class were admitted with me, the other students who were not admitted to the University because of lower grades, were successfully admitted in different universities all around the world for they all passed the general secondary examinations and with decent results. All 45 high school colleagues ended up in some sort of higher university education spread around the world.

The road to medicine was a very long, hectic journey. Usually it was two years of pre-clinical where the students study anatomy, physiology and biochemistry. The additional four years were where the clinical education kicks in with lectures and hospital rounds on a daily basis in all modalities of medicine. For six years, the student had to score passing grades according to the curriculum structure of the Royal Colleges of Physicians and Surgeons of Edenborough and Ireland. Curriculum, rules, regulations, exams and external examiners were all from England and Ireland. British professors came as visiting professors and all the local doctor teachers were educated and trained in the different modalities and specializations from English, Irish and Scottish hospitals and Universities and Royal College members. In the pre-clinical years, all professors had their PhDs from British Universities.

The six years of medicine together with the general science qualifying year took nearly nine years to complete. The military government was cracking down on university students for their protest against marshal law and seeking democracy. There was nothing called freedom to protest in a military government. The only way to stop student protest was to shut down the university classes and close the doors of the University sending students to their home towns and villages for students used to live in dormitories. The military government closed the university four times with different durations. I never got involved in aggressive riots, though I joined some of my colleagues in demonstrations against the regime. I remember the tear gas that when sniffed makes your eyes very itchy and tearing with burning sensations in your nostrils. Wet rugs were the key to relieve discomfort. Of course, being young and strong, we never got arrested for we used to run away from the cracking military. In one incident, there was a protest planned at the faculty of medicine, I did not attend, and the military soldiers cracked down on the students meeting and lashed them with camel lashes which are hard with tapered edges used to tame wild camels. A strong lash will get blood from the skin. Many students were injured, arrested and imprisoned. After few months they were released. Things calm down and the University was allowed to function as an educational institute.

Pre-clinical years were straight forward with lectures in the early mornings and laboratory work in the afternoon. The clinical years were similar with lectures early morning and hospital teaching rounds in the afternoon. At that time, faculty doctors were not permitted to have private practices, so that gave us the opportunity to return in the evening with the professors and continue our rounds with exposure and follow up of the diseases' progression. Although the third world country was poor, they had socialized medicine and everybody had access to free medical care in the hospitals resembling and following the socialised British medical system. Medical care was supplemented by the government and foreign aid. The professors were very keen to teach us and supervise precisely so that we could develop clinical sense in diagnosing diseases. In the late seventies, the hospitals had only X-Ray and general laboratory testing for blood, urine and stools. We had a blood bank for supplying cross matched transfusions and specialised pathology/biochemistry labs which detect complex diseases. Being a tropical country, there was a huge scope of tropical diseases, infectious diseases as well as the common medical problems faced by people around the world.

After completing both the didactic and clinical training we graduated from the faculty of medicine as physicians with a bachelor's degree in Medicine and Surgery "MB.BS". This qualified us to practice as house officers who were required to complete a full year of internship with obligations of three months' work in Medicine, Surgery, Obstetrics and Gynaecology together with a three month elective in the modality of choice. After completion, the house officer is qualified as a full practicing physician and is graded as a medical officer according to the ministry of health scheme which was derived from the English health system.

Before starting the housemanship (internship in America), we had to go to the presidential palace garden where the government held a ceremony for all graduates to take the Hippocratic Oath. All graduates attend and we, the Christians, were held at the last row for there were Bibles on each chair while the majority of the doctors took the oath on the Quran for the majority were Muslims. No doctor is allowed to go to the workforce if he/she did not take the oath.

The Hippocratic Oath was historically taken by physicians in Greece and is the most widely known of Greek medical text. Originally physicians vowed to the different Greek Gods to protect the patients and not use their knowledge to hurt or assist in destroying life ranging from abortions to helping in ending life for individuals.

The Oath had been modified several times. The most significant modification came about in 1948 by the World Medical Association (WMA) and called the Declaration of Geneva. This document was adopted three months before the United Nations in 1948 adopted the Universal Declaration of Human Rights which provided the security of individuals. In 1964 the dean of the School of Medicine in Tuft University in the United

States, rewrote the Oath and omitted any relation to prayers, so it was non-essential to be sworn on Holy Books or in reference to God. This version is used till today in all medical schools that require their graduated medical students to have an oath on graduation. It is actually the different governments in the world that enforce the oath when physicians are licensed to practice medicine. Unfortunately, with the separation of Church and State, and the poor religious upbringing of people in the modern era, society ignores religion and its teachings and physicians are left without an alert consciousness in not doing harm. You often hear of physicians approving and helping people to take their own life, performing abortions, subscribing narcotics unnecessarily, trying to gain an extra dollar by performing unethical deeds, signing their names on reports and diagnoses that they are not sure of, and sexually abusing patients. At the start of my medical career, I had yet to learn about such dirty practices. My goal was to uphold The Oath bringing help and healing to those in need.

CHAPTER 3

The Reality of Practicing Medicine

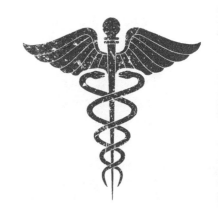

After qualifying as a physician, the journey for completing the housemanship (Internship in North America) year starts. It is a year of practice under supervision before being permitted to register with the country's medical council as a qualified physician who can obtain an unsupervised, unrestricted license to practice medicine. During the housemanship, the immediate supervision is from the medical officers who have completed their training and obtained an unrestricted license. The higher supervisor is the registrar (Resident in North America) who is preparing to qualify in the specialty of his/her choice. The consultant is the qualified physician who had obtained the membership of one of the Royal Colleges of Physicians and Surgeons of England, Scotland or Ireland.

The house officers are the first line of defense against disease. They run the hospital emergency departments of all specialties under the coverage of the medical officer and the registrar. The latter, besides supervising the house officers, have the responsibility of the inpatient wards, checking on all admissions and treatment schedules put in place by the house officer and the medical officer. All patients admitted on the day of the shift, will be the patients of the house officer who admitted them, and they are followed till they complete their treatment schedule and are discharged. The registrars have the responsibility of preparing the department rounds and in constant contact with the consultant in case he/she is required to attend to solve medical problems that could not be handled within the group. The registrars prepare the theater patients' schedule after consulting with the consultant and house officers, and, when they are not on duty, can attend operations and follow up with inpatients. In modalities where there are no operations, they participate in the outpatient clinics which are operated weekly. The house officers rotate in all department activities so they can gain experience and be prepared to enroll in any departments' activity when they are finally qualified to hold the place of the responsible party in the specialty of their choice.

There were two groups offering healthcare to the population. The majority of care was offered by the government hospitals under the supervision of the ministry of health and were spread all around the country. There was one university hospital linked to the Faculty of Medicine and all the staff supervisors are teachers in the university. The four major government hospitals were operated by consultants but rarely teach in the university. Only the very experienced are recruited by the university to help in conducting examinations in the different modalities as external examiners. They have especially strong links with the British external examiners who are invited to maintain international medical teaching standards.

There was a military hospital which is like veterans hospitals taking care of the military personnel and their families. The physicians and consultants staff of the hospital was all military personnel who trained as physicians before enrolling in the army. There was a tropical diseases hospital that was tending tuberculosis patients, for the disease prevailed in the country and the hospital was responsible for all tropical diseases. There was a specialized pediatrics hospital as well as a maternity hospital. As a result, the house offices had the option to enroll in any of these hospitals to complete their training. I elected to join the university hospital for most of my training in surgery and obstetrics and gynecology. I selected my special shifts in orthopedics for it was the most challenging with lots of shifts and exposure to emergency medicine. This, together with general surgery, will qualify the physician to become a surgeon if he elects that as a speciality.

The Housemanship or internship was the year that molds a physician to be ready for solo practice. I was lucky to have all the professors with whom I worked enforcing integrity, honesty, enthusiasm, superior patient care, dedication and execution of best practices.

Before starting my general medicine shift I was struck by a fever of unknown origin. Being unexperienced I sought the consultation of a family physician who was a family friend. For four weeks I had continuous very high fever that neither subsided by any antipyretic or medication given to me by the general physicians in town. On the sixth week, I was very debilitated, weak, and asked my uncle to take me to the university professor of medicine in his private clinic for he was my instructor and I had trust and believed in him.

I was escorted by my mom to go to the clinic, and while sitting in the waiting room, I suddenly started to see black dots in my field of vision and felt drowsy and lightheaded. I told my mom I started seeing black spots and I was not feeling good, she jumped from the chair beside me and rushed to the surgeon's office and told him of my symptoms. He left the patient he was interviewing came out of his office, went to the neighbouring internal medicine's office telling the professor inside that one of their recent medical graduates is seeing black and is drowsy in the waiting room.

Both professors escorted me to the examination couch. The internal medicine professor on examining me told my mom and my uncle that I was in very serious condition and was near death. He suspected enteric fever (typhoid) and ordered an immediate admission to the emergency medical department ward at the hospital. He asked my uncle to go find a wide spectrum injectable antibiotic from the private pharmacy since it was not available at the hospital. One of my uncles and my mom took me to the emergency department in the hospital along with other family members, while the other uncle went to get me the injectable medication.

From the professor's notes I was immediately admitted to the emergency medical department. There were no available beds and I was placed in a corridor in a bed that was made of local ropes, half of my body on the bed and half on the floor. The lights were very dim in the corridor and nurse on duty inserted an intravenous drip in my arm with the help of a family member's lighter to provide enough light. After half an hour, my uncle brought the intravenous medicine and when given to the nurse was injected into the intravenous drip and antibiotics were at last running in my system. When the first bag of saline and antibiotics was complete, my temperature eased off and I went to sleep as the rest of the medication continued.

This is the first time that I faced death knocking on my life's door; I never suspected that I could contact enteric fever from

The Reality of Practicing Medicine

the hospital wards where I was supposed to be training. I didn't believe that there were physicians, practicing there for years that could miss or even suspect the diagnosis of my unknown fever. Interestingly, one of the consulting general practitioners suspected it but failed to initiate a treatment trial. Because of this incident I was not afraid of death and determined, if I got well, to do my best to take advantage of my training and to be a very good physician. In the morning after my admission I was transferred to the university hospital where I spent four weeks under treatment and supervision of my professors, at the end I was released from the hospital after regaining my strength, and I thank God that I was alive.

After another month of home recovery I started my housemanship at the medicine department. As a house officer, one is responsible for the medical emergency department, the inpatients in the ward and the outpatients in the clinics where they were a subspecialty of hypertension and diabetes clinics, as well as tropical medicine clinics. Malaria, anemia, malnutrition, and gastrointestinal diseases were the main presenting cases. In the course of training to confirm cerebrospinal meningitis, we were trained to perform spinal tapping (insertion of a cannula in the lower spinal cord to get cerebrospinal specimens to the lab for confirmation).

By the end of my three-month training, I was called for a consultation one day to one of my relatives, they gave me the history that she ran a high fever for a couple of days and then lost consciousness, the private general practitioner in town was treating her as a diabetic coma and he was shooting in the dark for he gave her a glucose injection and she did not respond. After I examined her I suspected meningitis and told her brother and family that we need to take her to the general emergency department, for the physicians in the hospital would perform a spinal tap to establish my suspected diagnosis. Spinal tapping is a procedure where under sterile conditions a wide board cannula is inserted between the third and fourth lumbar vertebra of the lower back to access the spinal fluid, once the fluid starts coming out for collection if it is milky then the patient is sent to the quarantine awaiting the confirmation of the diagnosis. My relative's family refused my request of taking the woman to do such a procedure for they believed that there were cases where people got paralyzed from the spinal taps and specially none of the experienced practitioners suspect meningitis. I respected their wish noting to them if they are serious about her staying alive and regaining consciousness, I will help them to escort them to the hospital and advise my colleagues to perform the spinal tap to confirm the diagnosis.

After a few hours they returned to my house and asked me for my help since the lady never regained consciousness and they exhausted all of their resources. It was late afternoon when we drove her into the emergency medical department, I gave my colleagues the history and the suspicion of my diagnosis, they examined her and had the same suspicion of meningitis. They ordered the spinal tap kit to perform the procedure and obtain cerebral spinal specimen while I was in attendance with them. Once the spinal cannula was inserted, the trochula pulled out the spinal fluid. It leaked as a thick milky coloured solution establishing the diagnosis clinically and she was transferred to the quarantine to secure a bed awaiting the cytology results and anti-meningitis medication was started intravenously. When the results came it confirmed the diagnosis. After 24 hours of continuous treatment she regained consciousness and opened her eyes complaining of severe headaches that lasted for more than a week. Gradually she started talking and was lucky to not have any residual effects from the infection.

Obstetrics and gynaecology training was very interesting, bringing out realities that you will never find unless you are immersed in the practice, nearly 99% of all females were circumcised at that time, and it was very challenging to learn how to examine the female genital parts after such a procedure.

Female genital mutilation (FGM), also known as female genital cutting and female circumcision, is the ritual removal of some or all of the external female genitalia. This procedure is usually performed at an age varying from days after birth to puberty; in the countries where there are statistical data, the procedure is performed before the age of five. It is performed by a traditional circumciser who in most cases is an older woman (in communities where the barber is considered a health worker, he can perform the procedure; in some countries, more than 70% are performed by physicians) using a blade or razor with or without anesthesia, the younger the girl, the less anesthesia is used. It is common in many African countries, though it is also found in Asia, Middle East, and among different communities around the world.

The procedures differ according to the ethnic group. They include removal of the clitoral hood and clitoral glans (the visible part of the clitoris), removal of the inner labia and, in the most severe form (known as infibulation), removal of the inner and outer labia and closure of the vulva. In this last procedure, a small hole is left for the passage of urine and menstrual fluid, and the vagina is opened for intercourse and opened further for childbirth. Infibulation was adopted because it raised the price of female slaves in the era of human slavery. In some African countries, circumcision was modified to include breaking the front of the pubic bone. In some tribes, they fancy the procedure with removal of the clitoral hood, the clitoral glans, the inner labia and one side of the outer labia, then suturing the left part towards the removed part leaving a small hole for urine and menstrual cycles. This is performed to make sure that the girls do not have sex with any male out of the tribe for they won't know how to perform sexual intercourse.

The WHO, UNICEF and UNFPA issued a joint statement in April 1997 defining female genital mutilation as "all procedures involving partial or total removal of the external female genitalia or other injury to the female genital organs whether for cultural or other non-therapeutic reasons." WHO has created a more detailed typology that describes how much tissue was removed:

> Type I is subdivided into: I-a, the excision of the clitoral hood (rarely, if ever performed alone), and the more common I-b the complete or partial excision of the clitoral glans and clitoral hood (clitoridectomy).

> Type II is the complete or partial excision of the inner labia, with or without excision of the clitoral glans and outer labia.

> Type III (infibulation), is subdivided into: III-a, the excision and closure of the inner labia and III-b, that of the outer labia too. It is referred to as the "sewn closed" category, which are the excision of the external genitalia and the suture of the wound.

Type IV is referred to as "all other harmful procedures (pricking, piercing, cautering and stretching) to the female genitalia for non-medical purposes.

FGM can cause serious adverse consequences to girls' and women's physical and emotional health. Although it is fought and resisted in many countries as well as banned, unfortunately it is still illegally practiced in some parts of the world for religious as well as social obligations.

Ninety six percent of females were type III circumcised where you only find a tiny narrow opening at the perineum, the registrars told us how to perform a PV (paravaginal) examine and what to look for when reaching the uterine cervix. Gynecology was quite difficult when even trying to get a pap smear as well as swabs from around the cervix. When it came to obstetrics it was another nightmare for the babies are usually stuck in the birth canal where you need to do a lateral episiotomy to allow the advancing head to proceed, so the labour room was a horror theater where women were screaming and shouting during deliveries, doctors performing episiotomies, midwives helping a lot and receiving babies, nurses cleaning babies and helping them to get their first breaths. Though you can say it is a chaos inside the labour room where usually there were four females going into labour. It was a nightmare too for observing relatives who were outside the labour room. We, the physicians and the assisting groups, worked in harmony and made the best of the surrounding resources in delivering babies. The midwives had perfect training and were experienced to run most of the show.

I remember one time I was in the emergency room when a lady presented with gushing water and on examining her, found she was three fingers dilated. I felt something very stranger soft and mobile nothing like the babies vertex or face, on consulting with the registrar and he examined the lady and he told me that he did not know what that structure was and commented that the best person to identify this is the midwife in the labour room. We took her to the labour room, asked the midwife to examine the lady for she was in labour. On examination, the midwife burst into laughter and said, "hey doctors, you don't know what this is? These are the baby's testicles!" Of course we laughed too and performed a episiotomy where she delivered the breach baby buttocks first, then the legs, and the head was hanging down until the lower hairline was observed, at which time she put her hands between the vaginal opening and the baby's mouth and grabbing his feet pulling him towards his mom—a beautiful seven pound baby was born and of course the umbilical cord was cut and the placenta delivered. Just a note, that generally, we doctors used forceps to deliver the baby's head in breach deliveries. The episiotomy was sutured back in layers, and the lady was given an injection to reduce bleeding and to help contract the uterus. The placenta was placed in a bucket so as to dispose of it sanitarily. To my astonishment, I discovered that stray cats jumped into the labour room and stole the placenta to eat.

The emergency department was very busy; you can have twenty deliveries, fifteen D&C (dilatation and curettage), five to six C-sections (Caesarian Section) of obstructed labour and other causes. So, in the early morning hours one night after all this work and everyone was exhausted, I was called to examine a lady for whom, I was told, the baby was halfway out. I walked to the emergency department while all my colleagues (one other house officer, two medical officers and a registrar) were sleeping for we used to have a resting area with beds within walking distance. Before examining the lady, the nurse told me that the patient's mother asked for a female doctor, since that lady was a wife of the Imam (he is a person who teaches Islam at the mosque) I told her that we do not have female doctors on duty and from what I was told, if we don't examine her and try to save the baby, we might lose both of them and there was no need to tell the Imam any details. The mom accepted, as she realized her daughter's life was in danger.

When I examined the lady, I was shocked to find that the baby was a breach delivery, and somebody, delivering the baby at home, failed to do an episiotomy to deliver the head. On top of that, the umbilical cord was wrapped around the baby's neck and we had the baby's body hanging out from the birth canal and the head stuck in the mom's body. I ran and woke up the registrar who asked me if I was kidding for it was around 4:30 in the morning and the entire group was dead tired after a very long shift. With no other physicians to help, I told him that was what was really happening out in the emergency room. He examined the lady and determined that the baby was dead. He ordered the theatre for a C-section and we took the lady to the theatre where we performed the C-section decapitating the baby and removing the head from the uterus and removing the placenta and the body of the baby from the birth canal. He sutured the uterus and skin and sent the lady to the Obstetrics ward and that brought the early morning light where the next group physicians took over the emergency department.

The physicians on daytime rotation were from the university group, taking over for the ministry of health group who were on nights. On the morning rounds this incident caused a huge row from the university professors and they called the ministry consultant supervisor and told him that we had performed a procedure that has never been documented in Obstetrics practice history. We should have used the spear forceps to crush the baby's head, deliver it and clean everything out. The supervisor called us into his office where the registrar and myself informed him that the decision was made to perform a C-section for it was safer for the exhausted, drained woman, who might not have tolerated the crushing of the baby's head both physically and mentally, so in our discretion we figured out that the best scenario would be that what we had performed, taking into consideration all factors and saving the mom. The supervisor consultant praised us and told us that he would take care of the university professors. He called the professor and told him that his group was heroic in saving the mom and whatever procedure they performed was acceptable even if it had never been documented in Obstetrics literature. And so, after completing my three months of training in Obstetrics and Gynaecology I moved towards my next three-month rotation.

The General Surgery shift was shared between the Ministry of Health and the University. In the main city hospital, run by the Ministry of Health, we were working in the emergency department facing all surgical emergencies and admitting patients to the surgical wards. All operations and outpatient clinics were at the University hospital which was far away from the city centre. It had its own emergency department but since it was surrounded by villages and the population around the University hospital was small, it was elected to train physicians in the city hospital which is always busy.

This rotation shift trained us to be heroes. We labelled it as Heroic Medicine since we were trained to have superior clinical sense by diagnosing and immediately taking action to save lives. The only laboratory facilities available to us were plain X-rays and basic laboratory screening for white blood cell counts, haemoglobin and urinalysis. We were trained on diagnosing patients from history, complaints and physical signs aided by physical examination findings. There was no easy access to the consultants for the telephones were always out of order. In case the consultant is needed, we used to send an ambulance to their house. The registrars were physicians who were preparing to become surgical specialists and who have passed the preliminary examinations of the British Royal College of Physicians and Surgeons and are training to complete a practical curriculum with certain number of operations assisting the professors till they are able to operate alone. Once they had the skills of operating and managing a surgical department, they were allowed to sit for the final exams qualifying them to become surgeons. They were always available to us for consultation and possessed good skills and judgement that was passed to us thereby preparing our skills to enable us to handle the worst-case scenarios the surgical emergency department can accommodate.

On regular routine twenty-four-hour shift coverage, there would be 7-8 appendectomies, a few obstructed hernias and of course a wide scope of surgical emergencies from volvulus (twisting of the large intestine with obstruction) to spleen ruptures and stab wounds. The doctors running the surgical emergency department were moulded to be tough, courageous, and reactive with sharp diagnostic skills. They find themselves capable of diagnosing surgical emergency patients and executing treatment plans. That was tremendously important, for slacking, fear, or uncertainty will lead to patients' deaths. When they diagnose ruptured spleen due to injury from domestic fights, they immediately resuscitate the patient by placing an intravenous catheter with saline and send a blood sample to the blood bank for cross matching just in case the patient needs an emergency blood transfusion. The surgical theater and the anaesthesia team are informed to prepare for emergency laparotomy (opening the abdomen to explore the presumptive diagnosis).

The ambulance is sent to the consultant to inform him/her of the emergency. The house officer is the first line of defense, so he/she prepares all the afore-mentioned steps. The registrar and the medical officer supervising the day are immediately called in and almost as soon as the patient arrives at the theater, they start operating. Amazingly once the splenic vein and artery are identified and clamped with a non-crushing forceps, the blood pressure shoots to normal (it is usually very low showing signs of shock) and the anesthesia team adjust their anaesthetics till the operation is completed. During the laparotomy all abdominal organs are visually explored just in case there is another underlying problem. The abdominal cavity is cleaned up from any blood, the spleen removed, the peritoneum is sutured and the abdominal muscles sewed in layers. The patient is transferred to the ICU to start post-operative follow-up monitoring. When the patient is stable he/she is transferred to the surgical ward. I remember one of our surgical professors was always saying, "The abdomen is a magic box one can find any surprises inside. That makes laparotomy very challenging, like exploring the unknown." There were no fixed dates or timing for releasing patients from the hospital. When the surgical team clinically decide that the patient can resume daily functions, they order the discharge and release from the hospital with a follow up appointment in the outpatient clinic.

One of the striking incidences was a man brought into the emergency department very lethargic with a distended abdomen and severe pain. From the history and clinical examination, I suspected a volvulus (twisted large intestine). The plain X-Ray showed an inverted U-shaped colon with fluid levels. I prepared all the necessary resuscitation procedures: ordered blood cross matching just in case it is needed, called for the consultant, and together with the medical officer and registrar entered the theater to perform a laparotomy. The diagnosis was correct and I remember that for the first time in my training career I was about to vomit in the theater room. When we clamped the large intestine at the site of the torture, and cut off the gangrenous bowel, the smell that spread was like rotten contaminated human parts. That reminded me of the same smell during Forensic medicine training when we used to dissect lost people found dead for days in the outskirts of the city. The two ends of the large intestine were sewed together, the abdomen cleaned up, and the patient sent to the ICU.

One of our professors recounted to us an interesting incident in the history of medical discoveries. He said that the suturing of the intestines used to fail and patients die. One night the surgeon who used to suture the intestines, was sitting by the fireplace with his wife who was fixing his socks. He watched how she darned the ends of his socks after cutting through the hole. He thought of applying the same procedure to the human intestine; for at that time the standard method of joining intestine edges typically resulted in the death of the patient. Amazingly the procedure succeeded and the patient lived. From that day on, the procedure which was derived from darning socks became the lifesaving procedure for human beings.

In between emergency duties, which were the main purpose why we were under the emergency training elective, we followed the patients that were operated on by the surgeons in addition to the patients that were admitted during our emergency shifts, and sometimes we helped in the different surgical outpatient clinics.

Toward the end of my three months surgery training period, I used to operate on emergencies. I would prepare all patients who needed emergency surgery for the late-night hours of the shift, prioritizing immediate surgical needs followed by stable resuscitated patients. The emergency list was planned so as to be completed before seven a.m. since the theaters needed to be cleaned and prepared for all the cold cases scheduled to be operated upon the next day by the consultant surgeons. I used to run the surgical emergency all day. In the evening, I would typically send one of the nurses to purchase sandwiches for dinner under the condition that nobody eats till we finish the scheduled emergency surgeries.

Usually, we would eat in the early morning hours of the shift: that would be dinner or maybe breakfast. We would go wake up the tea man who starts preparing his kettle and supplies us with tea. If we completed our shift early we could go to the rounds to see the patients that were admitted and operated upon; otherwise we handed the surgical emergency to the next day group and headed home to get some sleep and rest. These shifts were repeated every third day for there were always doctor shortages. After completing the three months of the surgery shift, I proceeded towards my elective last three months.

My elective shift was in Orthopaedics (Trauma, in the western world). It was one of the most difficult electives to handle for it requires physical stamina as well as medical knowledge. I decided to indulge into the challenge for I was planning to proceed to Surgery as my future specialty. Electing this shift puts me in the track of becoming a surgeon. The experiences and training I gained from the nine months in the different departments eased the challenge I was going to face.

The Reality of Practicing Medicine

For instance, the training doctor is expected to run the emergency department for 72 hours straight. That means you have to be at the hospital for three continuous days of work with minimal coverage if ever needed, and this rotates every third day of the week. So you are working 72 hours in the emergency department, have three days of regular shifts at the wards, theater and fracture clinics, then back again to the 72 emergency shifts. There are no weekends or any days off to rest. You rest on the three days you are working in the regular shifts and in between quiet times in the rest area designated for doctors next to the emergency department. This makes the doctor available all times to trauma and emergencies. You are responsible for all traumas from simple wounds to open fractures (fractures of bone with wounds around fracture sites) in the whole city and the neighbouring regions. You suture wounds, reduce fractures, apply casts, clean dirty open fractures and prepare theaters for severe open fractures that need limb amputations. Amputations are the decision of the consultant surgeon and performed by the registrars. These experiences mould you to be a tough physician that can handle anything thrown at you.

There are lots of unforgettable incidences engraved in your memory when you work in such an environment. I will refer to the most unforgettable. In my early weeks of training, the ambulance brought in a labourer who was covered in dirt and unable to move. He was conscious but in pain. The history given was that he was in the 11th floor of a building under construction trying to remove a wooden mold from a concrete pillar. The wood snapped, and he dropped, flying to the ground. When his co-workers approached him, they thought they would find him dead. To the astonishment of everybody, they found him alive but unable to move.

On examination I detected that he had no voluntary movement of both his upper and lower limbs. He didn't feel a pin prick and his neuronal signs indicated an upper motor neuron lesion. In fact, it was determined that he had a fractured cervical spine which severed the spinal cord leading to quadriplegia. I confirmed the diagnosis with cervical X-Rays and admitted him to the orthopedic ward for further assessment and any recovery from the cervical cord shock.

I used to visit him regularly in my rounds when I was at the wards. After a few weeks we discovered that sadly we could not do anything for him to reverse the quadriplegia. His family was very supportive to him and had a dream that we, the doctors at the hospitals, would make him walk again.

A few weeks later, I remember being called to the ward to attend to another patient while I was on duty at the emergency department. That was during the afternoon at the middle of the visiting hours. The general orthopedic ward was large with about thirty patients' beds lying next to each other. After attending to the patient in need, I passed by to check on the quadriplegic patient for I hadn't seen him for three days while I was on my 72-hour shift. I greeted him and while talking with him, his sister jumped from her chair next to him and grabbed me by the neck shouting: "When is my brother going to walk again? He is here for more than 3 weeks."

I was shocked for she was watching very closely how her brother was taken care of and we were trying our best to prepare him psychologically for his tragedy. I didn't pull her hands off me but the nurses and the other visitors came to my rescue releasing her tight grip from my shirt around my neck. They called the police officer on duty at the emergency department after the people held her away from me. I told the officer that

I will not file any charges against her and later explained that she is emotionally disturbed because all his family members had the hope that we will make him walk again, unfortunately he will never walk again and we cannot do anything to help him in that regard. The officer, nurses, and some visitors talked to the sister and try to cool her down and to help her understand that the doctors were doing thier best for her brother. She later apologised to me.

Our consultant broke the news of no recovery to him and the family and that they would have to live with what they have; medicine cannot make miracles. After few months I was passing by the general surgery ward where I saw the same patient readmitted to the hospital. I went to greet him. He was very ill, lethargic, depressed, and very sad. I came to know that he was admitted with septic bed sores and was treated for septicemia. I wished him to be well and left. Unfortunately, this is a common tragedy for such patients in some areas of the world, they usually die from severe septicemia and nothing can be done for them. There are no specialized centres to handle quadriplegic patients and attend to their needs.

Another interesting and sad episode but with good outcome started when some people brought in a 48-year-old male patient in pain with a wrapped left lower limb that had a belt tightened around the middle thigh. The history given by the patient was that he was on his motor bike trying to turn around the roundabout when a truck hit him on his left side. He was thrown from his bike and the truck drove over his left leg. Passersby ran to his rescue and those accompanying him informed me that there was a lot of bleeding, so they had rushed to pull his belt out of his pants and tie it around his thigh to stop the bleeding. They said that there was a lot of dirt around his lower limb. They saw some bone and just wrapped everything in a rag and rushed him to the hospital.

On examination, he was stable clinically but in pain. I started an intravenous just in case things got worse and ordered blood cross-matching in case he would need a transfusion. He was moved to the small theater in the emergency department and I started exploring the wrapped left lower limb. On unwrapping the rag, I found out that all muscles around the fibula were torn off the bone and that there were neither muscle ends to connect nor skin to cover any anatomical parts. There were blood vessels hanging from both ends of the leg and it was very dirty with lots of ground debris. I cleaned the wounds by irrigating with normal saline and the registrar helped me to cauterise any visible blood vessels bleeding after we removed the belt tourniquet. In our opinion, the patient will need an above knee amputation. I wrapped all the tissue around the bone in sterile gauze and placed the limb in a posterior plaster slab keeping it straight. We immediately called for the consultant informing him of the emergency we had in hand.

Amputations are only performed after the consultant examines the patient and approves the procedure. Our debridement efforts were done under minor anesthesia and when the patient recovered, we informed him of our findings that the whole lower left limb was destroyed and there is nothing left for salvage of the muscles. After our consultant came to review our findings, he concurred that the patient would need an amputation to survive this unfortunate accident and proceed forward with his life using a lower limb prosthetic. The patient refused the idea and told us that he had an accident before and they had to fix his right knee. We informed him that he would be admitted to the general ward for observation and when our professor comes he will make the final decision. He was admitted to the general ward while we prepared all the necessary steps to proceed with the amputation operation.

When the professor arrived, we showed him our findings and he talked to the patient about an amputation operation. The patient refused an amputation and he was put on wide spectrum antibiotics and a follow-up regimen. The patient's family members were around him and supporting him, though in a week's time, he started to be lethargic, toxic and becoming confused. We informed him that all his misery would go away and he would recover if we proceeded with the amputation. In consultation with his family members and assurance that we will help him secure a prosthetic for his lower limb, he accepted the operation for he couldn't bear the agony anymore.

After the amputation he recovered very well and was discharged from hospital to follow up on the outpatient clinic. After few months while I was passing by the outpatient clinic, I saw him with a lower limb prosthetic and he hopped up from his chair, having a crutch on his right arm and came happily hopping to me, thanking me for all that I have done for him. I told him I was doing my job in helping people and was glad that everything went well for him.

One afternoon I heard the ambulance sirens outside the department and nurses were rushing children inside the emergency department. After the third child, I thought that a school bus had had an accident. Things were happening so fast yet I was able to discern that there were five kids, 3 boys and 2 girls, with an older woman, all brought in from the ambulance. I was told that no more patients were coming; I had all the injured. Lots of people came rushing into the department to see what happened, so I ordered the nurses not to allow anybody in and closed the emergency department doors since I was alone on the shift.

I found out that the dad hit the children and their mom on the heads with an axe. I quickly sent for help from the surgery emergency department and informed the neurosurgery doctors on duty. I quickly examined all the patients and found out that two kids and the mom were going into shock. I ordered the feet of the stretchers to be lifted and started an intravenous with the one who was worst. At the same time, I was looking for any bleeders in the exposed brains so I could ligate or compress. All patients struck on the right side had their brain exposed with hemiplegia, or paralysis, on the left side. Those struck on the left had hemiplegia on the right and their brain exposed there too. After starting the intravenous on the rest of the patients, I sent them, one at a time, for a skull X-rays, obtained blood samples for cross-matching and prepared all the admission files indicating the clinical findings.

The media arrived, as well as the hospital director was running around the emergency department. I left the door closed and had the situation under control. The consultant professor came to me asking what happened. He had access to the emergency room since he was responsible for the shift. I showed him all that I have done and that the situation was under control. He told me that he came because the hospital director called him and informed him that the emergency department was upside down and that there was no doctor on duty taking care of patients. I told him as you can see, everything was under control, all patients were resuscitated and safe, intravenous fluids were running, neurosurgery was informed and help was given from the surgery department to control the situation. All patients were controlled and they were sent to X-Ray with priority before proceeding to the neurosurgery theater. By now the neurosurgery personnel would be at their theater receiving patients. He was satisfied, congratulated me on my actions and left the scene.

Orthopaedics was so busy and hectic, but we enjoyed helping patients and saving lives. Our professor was very passionate but at the same time was specific and proud of his training doctors. When we used to reduce fractures and wrap them with plaster, he always insisted that the plaster should look smooth and nice so that whoever looks at the fixed limb will recognise that the reduction and plaster were done by his doctors under training. He was always available for consultation and always helped amputees to get prosthetics from the local limb manufacturers. The experience and training we received allowed us to handle any emergency situation wisely, patiently, and with superb positive outcomes. Although there were very limited resources, everybody was eager to do his best with whatever was available to save patients' lives.

CHAPTER 4

Discovering Unprofessionalism

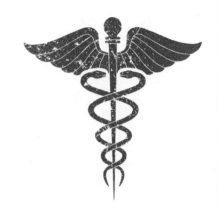

After completing my internship and qualifying as an unrestricted practicing physician, I was planning to go work in an Arabian Gulf country where lots of new technology was purchased and there seemed to be progression towards innovating the health systems by building new hospitals equipped from America and Europe with foreign leadership. My plan is to prepare for the FRCS (Fellowship of the Royal College of Surgeons) from either England or Ireland since these were the colleges that were supervising my medical education. So, working in the surgical field would equip me with the training duration required after passing the primary FRCS examinations.

I was naïve to share my plans with one of the Surgery registrars working with the ministry of health. I trusted him by telling him that we have relatives in one Arabian Gulf country who have very close friendship with one of our teaching professors working there at their University. I continued telling the registrar that I met with one professor when he was visiting and upon asking him to help me fulfill my plans, he informed me that if I gave his name as reference, I would be able to get a job in the field. He told me that he had arranged for one of his relatives to work there.

The registrar, knowing my plans, bad mouthed me to the supervisors to put me in trouble and prevent my departure to access an overseas job that would allow me to progress in the surgical field. I later came to know that he had the feeling and belief that when you graduate from your home country school of medicine, you should work in your own country and not seek overseas jobs to go serve other countries. Unfortunately, he was missing the point that staying in a poor, underdeveloped country would not give me the opportunity and challenge I was looking for.

The University where I got my medical degree was planning to separate from the English and Irish influence in education and try creating their own specialties with only very limited connection with foreign countries. That was a political move from the military government in spite of the fact that the British, when they colonised the country, had the upper hand in formulating all the basis of education in the university since they were the creators of the university, and after the country got its independence, they maintained the connection so as to keep the university linked to the universal standards of education. Nearly all professors had their qualifications from England or Ireland; some had their undergraduate qualifications from Arabic speaking countries. Of course beside politics, religion was playing a major part in formulating people's ideas and actions specially being the by-product of a colonised state. After independence, in the fifties, people hated the way the British was treating the locals but all the government and businesses were influenced by the British rules and regulations and the working class was disciplined to follow the rules.

On a later date, I found out that the professor working in The Arabian Gulf country lied to me. He had helped his Muslim relative to have a good job there and never followed on his promise to help me achieve my plans. In fact one of the teaching professors who like me very much told me that those Muslim Arabian Gulf countries do not welcome Christian doctors. Another professor close to me told me that my character is being honest and hardworking, and that definitely would not fit in the Arabian Gulf countries' system and I was better off going somewhere else.

Facing reality, I started thinking of an alternative plan. I will not be able to go work in the Arabian Gulf to facilitate the road towards specialising in Surgery. In my home country, I wanted to work as a medical officer in Surgery or Orthopedics but the ministry of health denied my preference and offered me a job in the Radiotherapy section. At that time in late seventies, the department was equipped with Radium generating equipment probably the first primitive form of generating radiation therapy for irradiating cancer. Unfortunately, 99% of patients die from radiation side effects rather than being treated from cancer. So that was a very depressing department where your work will be just completing medical records and preparing and signing death certificates. At that time, computers were not available, and all records are handwritten, and forms were submitted for completion. I declined the offer and resigned from the ministry of health.

I started to work on an alternative plan to continue my higher education and seek a specialty in Surgery. I have to pass the primary examination of the Royal College of Surgeons (FRCS). This was a test in Anatomy, Physiology, and Pathology. So, to have access to time and facilities, I planned to work as a demonstrator in the Anatomy department of the University meanwhile preparing for the part I examination. Once I pass the primary exam that qualifies me to work as a registrar who is under training to complete the required period before sitting for Part II of the FRCS. I was lucky that the Anatomy department needed demonstrators to help the undergraduate students with dissection and tutorials since Anatomy professors were leaving to the Arabian Gulf universities. The trend of doctors leaving to the Arabian Gulf was huge since they are paid good salaries and they are able to utilise the development that was happening on that side of the world. The departure of these doctors facilitated the hiring of new doctors to help the pre-clinical students, since their salaries were now available to be reallocated.

That was great news for me—I used to run a large section of the Anatomy dissection lab. At that time, we were teaching pre-clinical students on real cadavers; there were no plastic models there. The people, who were found dead, were brought to the morgue and lots of them had no relatives or next of kin to claim the bodies. It was very sad since the southern part of the country is a tropical jungle and people adventure to the North seeking better life, leaving their families and friends. They worked as servants and labourers in the North, being black and African, the Northern Arabs always treated and considered them as slaves, and locals usually called them 'Nigger'. So, there was an agreement with the Ministry of Health that the University may take for teaching, all dead bodies that had not been claimed. Every academic year one finds twenty-five to thirty bodies for students to dissect and learn from. The bodies, once received, are prepared by incising the jugular vein and artery connecting them to a formalin container circulating through the body for a couple of days replacing all the blood and cleaning all the organs, sterilising the body making it ready for dissection. The bodies are then submerged in a formalin basin and saved till the new group of students are ready to start dissection. When the school year starts, the students are divided into groups of twelve and each group is assigned a cadaver that stays with them for two years to complete the Anatomy didactic course.

People at that side of the world can be ignorant, naïve, and superstitious. One of the funny but sad incidences I remember happened when the morgue's night watchman began his shift one evening by walking into the lab. Suddenly, one of the bodies stood up from the basin. The watchman, consequently, ran away and lost his mind. The dead body was actually a worker taking a shower in the basin after they completed their afternoon shift of cleaning the newly built basin. He decided to take a bath in the clean basin before going home. The night watch guard was not aware there was work being done, and he thought that one of the dead bodies had come back to life.

At the end of the two pre-clinical years, all the bodies were actually only bones with little muscle attached, so the department used to clean the muscles and boil the bones, stripping them clean and making them available for students to study at the museum. I worked there for two years, dissecting about 50 cadavers and demonstrating to the students all parts of the human anatomy. In addition, I used to conduct tutorials and prepare the anatomy examination cadavers. Meanwhile, I registered for the local Part I Surgery qualifying examination at the University. So, my plan was working well. When the examination time approached, I was asked to prepare the cadaver for the Part I exam. The examiners were old Surgeons working with the Ministry of health as well as professors from the University. There were no British examiners.

I realised that the head of the department was marking my responses as wrong for selected parts of the cadaver, although I was the one who prepared the cadaver for the exam. When the results were released, we were thirteen doctors sitting for the exam, only two passed and they were the relatives of the professors conducting the exams. I realised that there was preference for relatives who were from the same religious and social status. That made me very angry and sad to find such unprofessionalism in conducting examinations and started to think of other options to fulfill my dreams.

My elder brother completed economics in the University. He tried to enroll in Medicine but his grades facilitated him to enroll in economics. He retook the higher Secondary School certificate exams for the second time while he was a first-year economics student at the university with the hope to score higher grades and change to General Science. When the results were released, he missed qualification by half a point, so he continued his education in economics and gave up the dream of going into Medicine. After he graduated, he had an opportunity to prepare for his masters and PhD at the University of Illinois in Chicago, USA. He was given a scholarship to go to America. When I asked him of any opportunities in the US, he told me that there is a course in Livingston, New Jersey that prepares foreign doctors for passing the ECFMG (Examination Commission for Foreign Medical Graduates).

That was an option that would open a great channel in the USA and I would be able to pursue my dream, continuing my education in the most advanced environment in Medicine. I started to make arrangements to leave for America. At that time, doctors were not allowed to leave the country, so I took a marriage leave and permission to go for a honeymoon. I took my wife and left for the USA seeking new adventure and opportunity. I stayed with my brother in Virginia since he had a job at a bank when he was preparing for his PhD.

CHAPTER 5

Discovering dirty Medicine in The USA

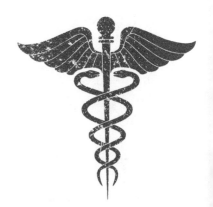

I arrived in America in February of 1982. My brother arranged for our stay in his home in Virginia. He had his mother in law living with him, his wife, and one daughter.

Snow was something new to me; I had only known it from the movies. It was nice to experience it for the first time—of course I had to get used to the winter clothing and having to wear multiple layers to go outdoors.

After a week, I left for Livingston New Jersey to register in the hospital where the postgraduate course for the ECFMG was going to take place. It was prearranged that I would stay in the attic of an old family using their daughter's room, as she was studying nursing in Delaware. This family was very sympathetic, generous, and very friendly.

I flew from Dallas airport in Virginia to Newark International Airport with the airbus was thirty-five dollars one way. The taxi charged fifty dollars from Newark International to Livingston.

In the first week, I met a doctor from India who was newly married and living in Virginia. He had a car and was driving to Livingston. We planned that over the weekend, we could spend time with our wives and then return to the hospital on Mondays. That was great! So we shared the gas and toll expenses since we used to take the New Jersey Turnpike, hitting the road for Virginia on Friday afternoon and returning back on Sunday night in preparation for Monday classes.

One weekend he asked me if we could leave Virginia in the early morning Monday so that we could drive straight to the hospital. I told him that it would be difficult to leave around four a.m. to reach the hospital for eight and continue a full day till five p.m. He said he wanted to spend more time with his wife and family. I accepted; he picked me up around three a.m., and we hit the highway.

Luckily, I can't sleep in anything moving, because after an hour on the road, I realised that the car was drifting from one lane to another and moving off of the road. I looked at my friend—his eyes were closed, indicating he was probably sleeping. I grabbed the steering wheel and yelled out to wake him up, asking him to stop at the side of the Turnpike. Although we used to take turns driving, I drove all the way to Livingston this time.

That night, I told him that I will continue in our agreement to go to Virginia every weekend under the condition that we leave on Friday evening and return on Sunday evening, otherwise our deal is off. It doesn't make any sense to risk our lives for the sake of a few hours per weekend; the course is only 3 months long and then we have all the time in the world to spend with the family.

Each day, we used to commute to the hospital from where we were living. A single mom with small car was trying to earn some money, so, she used to pick us up (four doctors all living in the area with other families) and drive us to and from the hospital for ten dollars each week from each of us. It was convenient, for the parking at the hospital was expensive.

The three-month ECFMG course, which cost me around US$7000.00 (keep in mind that was 1982), was taught by different lecturers on different medical specialties. Each lecturer used to train us on how to solve the multiple-choice questions since nearly all attending doctors had a different system of education in their home countries. I had the British system where the exam questions required written essays as responses.

One strange thing was mentioned by a lecturer during the first week of the Surgery class, , "In New York city there are 500 practicing surgeons who never attended medical school." When we asked for an explanation, he said that lots of American students go to the Caribbean Universities, spend five to six years enjoying themselves in the sun and on the beaches, pay for their education, and also pay the teachers, and then get a graduate degree in Medicine. When they come back to the States they are sponsored by either relatives or friends who teach them one surgical procedure; they get certified and start practicing the only thing they know. They cannot perform any other procedure since they are neither qualified nor knowledgeable enough to do so. That his statements held any truth was left to the listeners to decide for themselves. From what I have experienced in America, anything can take place, so what was stated could definitely be true. That was kind of disappointing to hear, for you work and study very hard to become the doctor you are dreaming to be, and other people just get what they want by paying their way through obtaining degrees and have relatives and friends that share in the shame of creating a profession for them.

After completing the course, I passed the ECFMG exams and thus qualified to apply for residency programs. I applied to as many programs as I could and actually secured some interviews. I came across one of my classmates who had studied medicine with me. He got married to an American girl and I came to know that he was doing his residency in Pediatrics with the ECFMG certification. I discovered later that his wife, being a nurse, he was able to obtain the residency through her, in spite of the fact that in the early eighties under Regan administration, the rules for foreign medical graduates had changed and they had to pass a visa qualifying exam before they could enroll in any medical training. That exam is nearly an impossibility to pass unless one has some experience in American hospitals for the American practice is different from most other medical practice around the world. I managed to stay in America for my wife got employed in an embassy and we were able to stay legally as people working in the diplomatic community. That did not give me the opportunity to secure any work in the medical field since medical practice was in the restricted list of employment for diplomatic family members.

While waiting for the residency program matching results to be released, I continued pursuing my dreams for Surgery by taking the FRCS Part I examination in Ireland and Scotland since I already had prepared for the exams once before in my home country. I continued studying in the public library, borrowed some money and actually registered to sit for the exams of the Royal College of Surgeons in Edinburgh and of the Royal College of Surgeons in Dublin. I flew to Dublin, stayed in a hotel and took the exams, then flew to Scotland where I had some relatives, stayed with them in Aberdeen then before the exam went to a hotel in Edinburgh to sit for the exams. I stayed another week with my family's friends to find out the results of the exams. I was disappointed when I came to know that on the British Isles, the exams have a political deviation. In Dublin, we were nine doctors sitting for the exam. One guy was a bright English doctor coming from Leads and he was the top of his class. All pointers were on him that he would pass the exam. Another doctor was an Indian working as a medical officer in Dublin and was sitting for the exam for the eighth time. An Arabian Gulf doctor, whose country gave him six years to pass the exam and this, was his second trial. The other doctors were, like me, travelling to sit for the exams. All doctors failed the exam with the exception of the Indian doctor who sat for the exam for the eighth time and another Irish doctor. That's it. Only two out of the nine doctors passed the exams.

Disappointingly, I didn't pass the Edinburgh exam either and didn't bother to check who passed and who didn't. I came to know that the British will pass you after you take the exam many times. A strange policy but that was the reality of the Royal College exams. I couldn't afford travelling to England or Dublin many times to sit for the exams. That trip alone cost me close to US$5000.00 as it was.

Subsequently, bad news came from back home. The military government had a very tight control and was cracking down on doctors and enforcing Sharia law as the law of the country. So, for me as a Christian, I would not be welcomed back even if I passed the Royal College exams. I convinced myself to forget about the Royal College exams and, already having a medical degree and permanent unrestricted registration with the medical council, I could enroll in my own private practice if I ever had to return to my home country.

Still pursuing the dream to join the American Medical system and obtaining my specialty, I contacted a doctor who had a prestigious position in an institution that was recruiting physicians from all over the world. I met him in my home country on one of his visits. He seemed to be a good person who encouraged me to seek options in America once we discussed my dreams towards specialization. I communicated with him and he worked with me to set up my resume according to the American system and highlight the points that show my strengths in medicine and the experiences I gained in working in different medical modalities. We designed a resume that was ready to be mailed to the different residency programs around the United States.

Sometime along the way, I noticed he started to act a bit weird, especially when he invited me and my brother to his apartment. The apartment was set up in a way similar to prostitute houses in Africa. He had dim light, wooden wavy curtains, and incense similar to what the prostitutes used in their places. He was wearing a galabia (one of the local dresses in African countries, made of a very transparent material that shows your body) and moving around his home. He offered us tea and brought to us a large book that had naked pictures of tribal people in Africa. He was a black person who told to us that he used to have good time when he goes to Africa with the men. He was indicating that he likes men, especially African men, and he is interested in having fun with sexual play. We did not show him any interest in what he was trying to do, politely spending some time reviewing his book and finishing the tea we were offered and left. We had realised that he is a homosexual trying to lure us into having a relationship with him.

We used to ignore such invitations from homosexuals in our country. We just don't get involved in such relationships for we are Christians and prefer women over men to have any sexual relationship. On my communication with him, he kept insisting on me having a relationship with him and plainly told me that

I should not ignore his desires. It came to a point that I wanted to get rid of whatever he is pushing me to get involved in, I told him bluntly that I am a married man and a Christian who does not get involved in sexual relations with men. It was our Christian cultural attitude to ignore gay men and that worked well back home since these people knew that we were not interested and we were left alone. This didn't work with this American gay doctor. He kept insisting on having a relationship for that will open the closed doors of Medicine.

When he realised that I would not break, he one day told me that since I was interested in women, there was a professor of medicine in a reputable university hospital. She was more than 50 years old and if I slept with her, she would help me to get my residency. I told him let me think about it and will get back to him so I could gain some time to figure how I could handle this situation.

That night I was sleeping next to my wife and couldn't sleep at all. The truth is that I didn't have any money, I didn't have a job, I didn't have anybody to help me; the only thing I had was my dignity, faith and self-esteem, and belief in God. I couldn't sell myself and loose the only thing I have for the sake of getting a job, having money and world prestige. I decided to tell that person off. Next morning, I called him and told him, "If you want to help me for God's sake to get my residency, fine and good, otherwise I can neither have a relationship with you nor with the older professor. I am a Christian, believe in God, married and never got involved in any relationships like that before and will never get into one now." He responded, "Fine it's your choice!" and he hung up.

When the matching program results were finally released, I didn't match in any of the hospitals I was interviewed in. One of the interviewers in Pennsylvania wanted me to send him to a safari in Africa to shoot lions and elephants in lieu of giving me a residency. I didn't have the money to do that and besides, that was inappropriate to obtain a residency in such a manner. It seemed that residency programs were offered to foreign medical graduates by subjecting them to pressure and satisfying personal greed from program directors and the persons in positions to offer jobs. So I called that gay black doctor and told him that I didn't match with any of the hospitals I was interviewed in. He responded in an inhumane, inconsiderate, unsympathetic tone, "You have to live with the consequences of your principals." I responded to him, "how can you sleep at night treating people like that?" He responded, "Oh! I sleep very well and nothing bothers me." I hung up and never called him again.

Let's tackle this gay and lesbian issue and under the freedom of speech, I will exercise my right to talk about this subject. People might disagree with me, but this is my personal belief and opinion, and I am not scared by any means by laying it out in the open.

When I was studying medicine in the seventies, gays and lesbians were listed in the psychiatric literature as patients who are mentally disturbed and need attention and treatment. Later, when the DMS III was published they removed this from the psychiatric literature and it is no longer considered a disease. Politics played a huge part in the evolution of the movement and human rights commissions were influenced to treat these people as deprived, discriminated against and laid out rights and privileges so that this community may exercise a way of life that is not acceptable to all religions around the world. Being a Christian, I will tackle this issue from a Christian point of view in which I share and believe. In the New King James Version of the Old Testament, in the third book of Moses, Leviticus, where the basics of life are laid down by the Lord our God and many of the rules are exercised in all countries around the world, the LORD spoke to Moses instructing him about the forbidden immorality in Leviticus 18:22:

> "You shall not lie with a male as with a woman. It is an abomination."

In the same book, the LORD laid the moral and ceremonial laws, in Leviticus 20:13:

> "If a man lies with a male as he lies with a woman, both of them have committed an abomination. They shall surely be put to death. Their blood shall be upon them."

In the New testament, in the Epistle of Paul the Apostle to the Romans Chapter 1: 24-32:

> 24 Therefore God also gave them up to uncleanness, in the lusts of their hearts, to dishonour their bodies among themselves
>
> 25 who exchanged the truth of God for the lie, and worshiped and served the creature rather than the Creator, who is blessed forever. Amen.
>
> 26 For this reason God gave them up to vile passions. For even their women exchanged the natural use for what is against nature.

27 Likewise also the men, leaving the natural use of the woman, burned in their lust for one another, men with men committing what is shameful, and receiving in themselves the penalty of their error which was due.

28 And even as they did not like to retain God in their knowledge, God gave them over to a debased mind, to do those things which are not fitting;

29 being filled with all unrighteousness, sexual immorality, wickedness, covetousness, maliciousness; full of envy, murder, strife, deceit, evil-mindedness; they are whisperers,

30 backbiters, haters of God, violent, proud, boasters, inventors of evil things, disobedient to parents,

31 undiscerning, untrustworthy, unloving, unforgiving, unmerciful;

32 who, knowing the righteous judgment of God, that those who practice such things are deserving of death, not only do the same but also approve of those who practice them.

In the Epistle of Paul the Apostle to the Romans Chapter 2:1-2:

1 Therefore you are inexcusable, O man, whoever you are who judge, for in whatever you judge another you condemn yourself; for you who judge practice the same things.

2 But we know that the judgment of God is according to truth against those who practice such things.

In the First Epistle of Paul the Apostle to the Corinthians Chapter 6:9-11:

9 Do you not know that the unrighteous will not inherit the kingdom of God? Do not be deceived. Neither fornicators, nor idolaters, nor adulterers, nor homosexuals, nor sodomites,

10 nor thieves, nor covetous, nor drunkards, nor revilers, nor extortioners will inherit the kingdom of God.

11 And such were some of you. But you were washed, but you were sanctified, but you were justified in the name of the Lord Jesus and by the Spirit of our God. Glorify God in Body and Spirit.

    I have no problem with gay and lesbians individuals. They have their own lives and they can do whatever they want and I neither suggest nor tell them how to live their lives and this is part of living in the free world as we know it.
    The problem I have with these people is when they force themselves to use their sexual desires to obtain self-satisfaction by inflicting themselves on vulnerable individuals who are seeking help to survive in the world. The gay and lesbian community should refrain from such actions and respect the dignity and beliefs of other individuals living around them. It is a human rights violation when they impose themselves on innocent individuals, who are trying to survive the difficulties of life, for

obtaining their own sexual self-satisfaction. At a later date, I found out that the gay doctor was part of a large professional group whose members are spread around the US. The group have the ability to recruit doctors from all over the world, bring them to the United States, getting them involved in their personal sexual satisfactions and helping them to obtain residency programs. Those victim doctors become sexual slaves for the professional group for whoever needs any sexual satisfaction will go to them and on top of that, they obtain portions of their income as security for not exposing their actions. What a dirty pathetic way of practicing medicine.

CHAPTER 6

Terrible Experience of Medicine in the Arabian Gulf

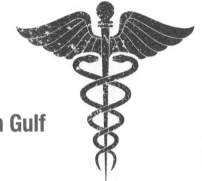

After living through in the experience of trying to obtain a residency and specialty in the United States, I decided to seek going to the Arabian Gulf again. Still having the dream to pursue higher education and specialization, I was applying all around the Arabian Gulf countries to obtain employment that would help me earn some money and at the same time pursue my dreams in medicine. I got a job offer from a small country in the Arabian Gulf I was so excited that directed all my efforts to go there and explore the dream of working there and obtaining my specialty. My wife had secured a job in an embassy in the US as a secretary, so I left her there and flew to the Arabian Gulf.

After a twelve-hour flight connecting through Heathrow airport in England, British Airways landed in the country's airport. I encountered something quiet peculiar: there were signs all around the airport warning travellers that photography is prohibited. It was astonishing for there was nothing to take pictures of. It was a flat clear desert as far as your eyes can see.

We were instructed not to leave the plane. Somebody came up to the plane and asked for our passports took them and informed me that I would be escorted to a hotel once I disembarked from the plane and obtained my luggage.

I took my luggage and went through customs. I had sixty kg of books with me; the inspector asked me if I was a teacher or a doctor. I told him these books are my references for doctors use them as references when practicing. I was escorted to a hotel in the late afternoon. The hotel was nice; the room was cooled with an air conditioner.

I wanted to freshen up by taking a shower after the long flight. When I put the cold water on, steaming hot water came out of the shower. I tried all valves, and it seemed that there was no cold water in the shower. I called for the bell boy and when he arrived, I asked him if there was something wrong with the shower as there was no cold water. He asked me where I was coming from, I told him from America, he laughed and told me that this was the water coming from the taps on the top of the hotel water tanks. At this point, there was no cold water; although, the hotel was in the process of installing tanks that would cool the water and then there will be hot and cold water in the taps. So, I took a very strange shower: I went under the hot water until I felt very hot, then ran to stand in front of the air conditioner. This process continued until I finished showering. What a shower experience!

Next morning, somebody came and escorted me to the hospital I was assigned to. The trip took five hours from the capital. The entire road to the hospital was all desert and mountains; there was no sign of life anywhere. On reaching the hospital, I had the shock of my life. The hospital was a one floor building with a fence around it and two large entrance gates, not at all what I was expecting for a Gulf Country where medicine had a reputation of being cutting edge. In addition to that, it was in the middle of nowhere, you could see only desert all around and the mountains on the periphery.

I met with the local medical officer who told me that I would stay in the residence adjacent to the hospital. I was helped by some Indian workers there to take my luggage and go to the residence. Upon entering, I found it to be a two-bedroom apartment with a kitchen and bathroom. It was furnished with a bed, dresser with a mirror, a dining table with few chairs, a couch and a chair. The bathroom was the most disgusting place I had ever seen in my life. I had to walk to the hospital at once and asked if there were any cleaners that could help me clean the place. I was able to secure the help of the hospital cleaners, asking them to please clean the apartment for me, especially the bathroom and I would pay for the time they spend there.

By midnight the place was clean and livable. I put my suitcases into the bedroom and, being very tired, wanted to take a shower. Unbelievably, the water was so hot at midnight, but I managed to take a shower and all the time I stayed there, I would shower at midnight for the water was even warmer during the day than midnight. I also think water was quite hard, for after a shower, white deposits remained on my skin even after drying myself with a towel. I didn't have any choice, I had to live there, so I adapted as much as I could.

The next morning, I was introduced to the hospital staff. They were all Indian doctors who didn't speak a word of Arabic, except one who spoke Arabic because he had worked there for 5 years. The local medical officer He told me that there was a small village close by where I could buy my food and that most of the doctors were staying in a nearby building and were transported to and from the hospital daily by a mini bus. There was a small private grocery store next to the hospital that was owned by an Egyptian.

The medical officer informed me that my salary would be US$900.00 a month and it would be deposited into a bank account. The salary was a disappointment to me; I thought that I would have been paid US$2000.00 per month taking into consideration the four years of experience I had practicing medicine. With no tax and free residence, that would have been not a bad wage for some time.

There was an oncologist running the surgery department, an anaesthesiologist helping him, a female gynaecologist, an internist in medicine and all the other doctors were general practitioners. They lacked any emergency medicine expertise, so since I was the only one with trauma experience, my services would be a huge asset to the hospital for it was located in an area that covers a very dangerous bend in the road going to the United Arab Emirates and there are, as a result, many car accidents in addition to the trauma from the nearby village.

Our duties were scheduled in such a way that each of us covered the emergency department for twenty-four hours every fourth day. The rest of the week, we covered the outpatient clinics. I was astonished that the Bedouin (desert people) would come to the hospital for entertainment, to check out the new doctor arrivals.

Since, the Indian doctors did not speak Arabic, they did not understand what the patient was complaining about; they would listen, examine the patient, and then write a prescription of medicine. The patients then go to the pharmacy to order the prescribed medication, look at the tablets, taste the tablets, and if they had taken them before and they didn't work, they would throw them out in the trash which were two large drums on each side of the hospital gates. What a waste!

The locals daily came to the hospital, bringing their coffee, food and dates and kind of picnic in the hospital under the palm trees. In the Arabian Gulf, the people drink coffee in a special way. The cups are small, filled halfway with warm coffee, and every time they take a sip, they eat a date; they do not use sugar for the coffee.

The chief medical officer is an Indian doctor who speaks Arabic. He was there for a long time, and he wouldn't hesitate to operate on any emergency from appendicitis to duodenal ulcer ruptures which were the most common surgical emergencies that patients present due to the common eating habits of the workers from India and Sri Lanka. The nurses and midwives were all Indians and the only local employee was an outpatient clinic door keeper organising the flow of patients. Amazingly, I was told that he is paid the equivalent of US$3000.00 salary each month being a local employee.

The environment was nothing close to what I had expected going in. There was no cafeteria in the hospital, so you had to cook your own food. To obtain food, you needed to go to the village stores. One of the doctors had an old car which is functioning, but the sun and heat had nearly stripped all the paint off the top, even though he parked it under a straw shed somewhere in the hospital compound. He drove once a week to the village market to purchase whatever was needed. He also helped his colleagues by taking them to purchase groceries from the market.

All doctors were transported to and from the hospital with a minivan belonging to the hospital. They were brought in at nine a.m. and returned at five p.m. I was placed in the small apartment close to the hospital for I was the most experienced physician in the hospital with trauma training and could offer emergency treatment. The working conditions were terrible and I didn't see myself surviving for long in that environment. One of the nurses told me that at the Sultan's area, his staff and immediate family hit the doctors with slippers on their head if they are not satisfied with the treatment they get. This is the highest insult at that side of the world.

After two weeks, I requested a meeting with the undersecretary of the ministry of health in the capital. I went and met him to submit my resignation. He questioned me on why I came to join their service. I told him that I was coming to serve the sick meanwhile preparing for my FRCS (Fellowship of the Royal College of Physicians and Surgeons) to specialize as a surgeon. He asked if he could transfer me to the Sultan's area hospital, would I accept working there. I told him if he could guarantee me working in the surgical department, I would accept the transfer. He replied that he couldn't guarantee anything and I could be moved to any place in the country at any time. So, after only two weeks' time, I submitted my resignation to shorten my compulsory one year contract agreement to work only a three months duration, the end of which time they would give me back my passport and allow me to leave the country. For simplicity, I asked to be kept in the original place I was assigned, for I was settled there and more than that, my services were needed in that area for none of the staff had any experience in handling emergencies and trauma. He agreed and I returned to my assigned hospital.

Food was a problem for me. I went with the doctor who had the car to the village market, and only bought instant noodle soup. The contents must have been bad, for I got food poisoning: I had severe diarrhea and vomiting. I sent somebody to the hospital to get one of the doctors. When he examined me and had my history, he told me that it was indeed food poisoning, and those instant soup noodles probably were expired for nobody eats them there. I got some medication and drank lots of bottled water. Then I took all the noodles I had bought and threw them in the garbage. After which, I arranged with the store keeper in front the hospital to bring to me on weekly basis: a dozen eggs, a case of Pepsi, a case of water, three boxes of crackers and canned yellow cheese. So, after the food poisoning, I started to eat two eggs with a piece of cheese and some crackers. Hydrated myself with water and Pepsi and drank tea in the morning and afternoon. I lost sixty pounds in the three months I stayed there.

I covered all emergencies in the hospital. I was glad that I submitted my resignation to shorten the time of my stay. I came to know that foreign workers are treated like slaves. In one incidence, an Indian worker was brought to me with tibial fractures of both his lower limbs. After examining him and before I started to treat him, the door keeper came to me and told me that this patient is not covered under the ministry of health and since he is on a private contract with an individual, he has to pay sixty Riyals, thirty for each lower limb. In my history taking for the accident, the patient told me that while he was preparing the big stone which compresses the bricks they are manufacturing, the stone slipped and fell on both his legs causing the fracture. One of his fellow workers who brought him to the hospital told me that the owner treated the workers in such a way that if he found anybody sleeping, he is deported the next day to his country and his contract terminated. The workers prepared a hedge where they took turns sleeping behind it so they don't get discovered and fired. He told me that they are paid thirty Riyals (around US$90.00) for a whole month's work. So, for this patient to get treatment to get his fractures reduced, he would have to pay two months' salary and he would be sent back to his home country for he can't work till his legs heal and he can start walking again. I told the door keeper that this patient is going to be treated for free for he cannot pay for the treatment and we have to be human and consider his circumstances. I told him, if anybody raised any questions, they have to come and talk to me.

So with that, I began my treatment on the patient. After giving him a sedative for the pain, I asked him to sit at the edge of the examining table with both his lower limbs hanging down to allow gravity to reduce his fractures. When the muscles relaxed, and the lower limbs were more or less straight, I prepared plaster and reduced the fracture while rolling the plaster around the limbs forming a below-knee fixation to his fractures. My successful reduction was confirmed by X-ray. Thus, I placed the man in a wheelchair, gave the X-rays to his friends, and asked them to return him back to his country for his contractor will deport him anyways. I treated the patient for free for it was unfair to collect any fees from a patient with very low wages, and besides, there was so much waste by the locals who threw their medications in the hospital garbage bins.

In addition to my regular work in the emergency and outpatient clinics, I used to do rounds in the hospital beds and check on inpatients whom I have admitted, or others admitted by other doctors. You are not allowed to go near the Obstetrics and Gynaecology ward. Only the female gynaecologist and the female nurse are allowed in those wards. It was very difficult to treat any female patient who was involved in an emergency; they just don't want male doctors to examine or treat their females. In fact, one time they brought me a female patient who was running high fever and nearly unconscious. When they discovered that I was the only doctor on duty to examine her, they took her back and I couldn't examine her. As far as this is weird, their religion prevents their females to be exposed to male doctors and if the patient dies, it doesn't matter.

On another occasion, there was a local old man who was married to two women, an old local lady and a young Egyptian woman. The latter told me that the family hated her, and they did not want her to have any inheritance when the husband dies. The old man had fractured lower spine and was paraplegic. He was diabetic and had a heart problem.

I tried to help this old paraplegic patient by sending him to the capitol for consultation on his case and how we should handle it. They returned him back to us telling us that they could do nothing for him more than the medication he was already on and that we had to continue palliative treatment under our supervision.

After 2 months in one of my evening rounds, I saw his bed empty and when I asked about him, I was told that he had passed away. I questioned how that happened for he was doing well the day before. They told me that his family brought blood from the UAE and when he was given the blood he passed away. I investigated this story and went to the blood bank to ask about what happened. I found out that the family brought two pints of blood they gave him one and the other was still in the fridge. When I shook the leftover blood pint, it made foam, so probably the blood was expired. I called the chief medical officer and showed him how the blood pint foamed and I told him that the family brought expired blood and that killed the poor old patient. He just shook his head and left. I didn't pursue this for it was not my responsibility to follow the case any further. I disclosed the facts and it is up to the management to follow up. On that side of the world, you can purchase blood from any neighbouring countries, unfortunately there is no way to check on the validity of the obtained blood and there were no rules and regulations governing such actions.

In another incidence, an Egyptian teacher came rushing into the afternoon outpatient clinic coughing and puffing and demanding that I do an X-ray for his chest. I was very popular around the teachers at that time since I was practicing medicine honestly and when patients come under my care, I took a good history and subjected them to proper investigations to reach to a diagnosis. I discovered lots of patients with diabetes, with high cholesterol, and high blood pressure. All newly diagnosed patients were treated accordingly, and I managed to explain to all of them what their diseases were and to give them advice about food and lifestyle changes.

When examining the Egyptian teacher, I found that when he lay flat on his back with his head straight on the table, he turned red and choked and I had to quickly put him in the sitting position and immediately sent him to X-ray. When I checked the X-ray, I didn't find any heart borders; actually there was a rounded ball of shadow in the heart area between the lungs. The lungs themselves were clear. The first thing I thought of was that it was an X-ray artifact. So, naturally, I requested a repeat X-ray, yet the same results came back with a ball shadow in the heart's place; the rest of the fields were normal.

I called the internist and when he examined him, he too was puzzled. We didn't know what is going on, so the best way to obtain a definitive diagnosis was to send him to the capitol where they have specialized hospitals. I arranged for an ambulance to send him for consultation. It was deemed necessary for the consultants to do a chest exploration to detect what that strange anatomical structure was. At that time they didn't have CT scans or MRI to detect any abnormality. The patient was normal except for this finding and that when he lays flat, he chokes. The patient got scared when the hospital asked him to sign a consent form so they could do the exploratory thoracotomy. He refused any surgeries and returned back from the capitol.

He came to me and consulted with me, bringing along his wife, young daughter, and his six-year-old son. I told him I suspected an aortic aneurysm that could rupture at any time, so he was better off doing the exploration so that a diagnosis could be established and if there were any treatments, he would have them. It was a hypothetical diagnosis since, as I stated, at that time medical imaging was not yet advanced and there no imaging devices. I told him to be a strong believer and ask God to help him and his family. There was nothing to be scared about and if he was going to die, he would die of any other cause beside his medical unknown problem. They accepted my advice and he planned to go back to the hospital and sign the consent forms and proceed with the exploratory surgery.

I called the thoracic surgeon who was going to perform the operation and told him that the patient is going to sign the consent forms and that he will be ready to find out the mystery of the swelling. After the operation, the surgeon called me and gave me a verbal report: he had found a coconut shell sized tumor on the pericardium covering the heart. That was what was blocking the heart contours in the X-rays, and on opening the shell, the fillings were confirmed by pathology to be a sarcoma, one of the rarest tumours you can ever find in that area of the body.

After the surgery, the patient returned to his family all smiles and happy. As a virtue of thanks, the family brought a gift for me and asked if they might borrow the condo keys so they could leave it there for me. I gave him the keys, thanked him and told him that I really didn't want anything: I was doing my job and was glad that everything worked out well in the end. When I returned to my apartment, I found a metal cookie box in my bedroom. When I opened the box, I found a gift of a baked chicken and roasted potato. Remember that I hadn't eaten for more than two and half months! I ate and then divided the chicken into portions that lasted me a week. That was really nice of them, I needed that break. I tried to send the patient to Saudi Arabia where he could be followed up and if there was any need for chemotherapy, he could obtain it there. The ministry of health refused, telling me that he was an expatriate and had no right to be treated abroad. He had a few months left before the completion of his contract. I advised him to complete his contract, take whatever he is paid and then leave to Egypt. There he can consult with the Egyptian doctors and if he would require any radiation or chemotherapy, he would get it for free.

At last my three months in the desert were complete and I was ready to head back to the United States to join my wife. I recall the last day I stood up on a small hill with goats running around me and looked around to the sand and mountains and told myself that I stayed three months in hell and couldn't get used to the environment. I thanked God that he allowed me to go back to my pregnant wife in America. I was going back with no plans and no ambitions for that experience had a huge toll on me physically and mentally.

CHAPTER 7

Discovering real dirt in the American Medical System

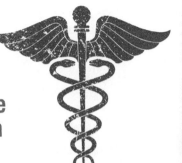

On my return to the States and after I recovered from the crisis I passed through in the Arabian Gulf, I found a part time medical translator job with the Arabic speaking embassies to translate for the patients seeking medical care in America. My wife still held the receptionist job in an embassy. Some Arabian Gulf embassies have medical offices that are administered by doctors qualified overseas but cannot practice medicine in America. Those established medical offices never gave me a chance to join their staff for they prefer Muslim doctors over Christian doctors. Anyways, I offered my services to the other embassies that get patients from overseas and needed a translator. So, whenever there was a chance, I was available to help, although with only minimum wage per hour. Two unforgettable shocking incidences are worth mentioning.

An Arabic speaking obstetrician and gynaecologist had most of the patients referred to him. That doctor knew that I was translating to the sheikhs and patients who came from the

Dr. Nabil Basanti

Arabian Gulf and that I was looking for my residency. (Of course, I only accompanied the males for females are not allowed to be accompanied by males and they had other female interpreters.) He had access to a hospital where he could follow his admitted patients, and although he suggested that he could offer some help in securing a residency position for me, he had no power to do so.

He had a ninety-year-old sheikh who was married to a nineteen-year-old girl from another royal family. The sheikh wanted to have a child with his young wife but he was unable to make her pregnant. The obstetrician told me that we could help the sheikh by impregnating his wife with my semen. He told me that my features were Arabic and they would never find out. He offered me US$400.00 for my semen. I was shocked when he asked me that. I told him that would be adultery for the baby would be mine and I couldn't do something like this even if he paid me thousands of dollars. It's a matter of principle and not money, we could do artificial insemination with the sheikh's semen, if there were any live sperm in his semen, but that would be the proper way to do it. He told me that the sheikh would find that an insult and so, it wouldn't work. At a later date, I found out that the gynaecologist was using this method to make the young wives pregnant by inseminating them with other people's semen and charging the sheikhs US$100,000.00 per pregnancy. What a way to practice medicine! This gynaecologist had a very bad ending; he was a nervous person and had problems in dealing with people. His daughter testified against him when her mom died because he pushed her down the stairs during an argument. He is serving a life sentence in jail for he was found guilty of murder.

The other unprofessional, disgusting, dirty practice was when one sheikh needed a kidney transplant. There was a professor of urology in a reputable university hospital that arranged kidney transplants by offering a kidney for US$250,000.00 and with the hospital stay and operative costs and recovery, the total cost would be close to a million US dollars. The astonishingly strange thing was that Americans had donated those kidneys with the understanding that they be made available for Americans who were on dialysis, waiting for a kidney transplant. So, the sheikhs, coming from overseas, by way of money and greed, skipped the line and secured kidney transplants depriving those poor American patients, legitimately on the waiting list, and forced them to continue on dialysis denying them a chance for a kidney transplant. On a later date, I found out that they arranged prostitute nurses to serve the sheikhs in recovery so that they could have sex, proving to the sheikhs that they are perfectly normal after the transplant and thereby could return to their homeland to enjoy their life. That was an important assurance for those patients since sexual activity is mandatory for proof of being healthy. The hospital and the professor performed many such transplants for patients coming from overseas.

Being completely disappointed in the medical environment in America, I started to lose interest in joining the system to obtain higher education and specialisation. Thankfully, I managed to get a job in health insurance administration in one of the embassies. They had an office that took care of the educational needs of the students and their families. The program was huge and there was lots of talk about the health program they were administering through the embassy. I met with the first secretary who offered me the job to try to control the cost and to supervise the medical needs and health of the students and their families. During the interview, I came to know that the health insurance program cost the country US$ nine million for 3500 students, some of whom were married and were dispersed all around the States in different universities. He gave me the results of an audit that was performed by a private health auditor he had hired. He informed me that he was leaving his post in the embassy and that nobody had access to the audit and that I should use it to correct the problems they were encountering in the administration of the health insurance program and make things better for the students. He trusted me and told me to share the audit with neither the senior nor the junior embassy employees.

I was given a desk in the open area where all staff working with the students were located. There were dividers between staff for some privacy. There was one employee already working in the health insurance program with an accounting background and a secretary who was advised to help me in secretarial work. That employee spoke Arabic, so he was able to communicate with the students and had some connections with the main embassy senior staff. Before I was hired, they had a broker who was administering the program through a reputable insurance company. The insurance company advised the embassy to remove the broker and to work directly with them for administering the students' health insurance program. Through a series of meetings, I made a good relationship with the different departments of the health insurance company. Now, being the manager of the health insurance program, I assigned the person who was already working there to have limited managerial activity and he was restricted to only check on student's validity to join the program, register them, and issue health insurance cards through the enrollment department of the health insurance company. I took over all the managerial decisions, planning, and execution of the health insurance program.

The group of students expected the same social medical privileges that they enjoyed in their home country. Whenever they would seek medical care from a doctor or specialist, they booked an appointment, and after the visit, the doctor or specialist would bill the insurance company and the insurance company then paid the bill. So, the insurance company was retained to process payments without restrictions. This, of course, would not work to the doctors' benefit and would end up costing the consumer a lot of money. I reviewed the benefits the students were offered. I rewrote the American benefit health coverage to fit the socialised health benefits the students expected. The student group was made aware of the rewritten health benefits and was encouraged to follow the new methodologies in obtaining treatment for whatever sickness they encountered. On the other hand, I was administering a student health program whose population was between the ages of eighteen and twenty-five, so supposedly they would be healthy and should not cost the government millions of dollars for health benefit coverage.

Working with the statistical department at the health insurance company and being under diplomatic immunity coverage, I was able to obtain through the legal department, the health utilization profile of the covered student population. Piles of computer printouts were delivered to my office with stacks of paper one meter high from the floor to the top of my desk. I literally went through all the stacks of computer printouts, page by page, analysing the utilization of the health benefits I was administering. My request for the utilization break-down was by student ID number, utilization by category, usage and cost.

I discovered catastrophic treatments offered to our students by the American doctors. There were huge numbers of cholecystectomies (gall bladder removals). There were many accounts of hysterectomies (removal of the uterus) for young female students, as well as a plethora of mastectomies (removal of breasts). I couldn't believe that these were genuine operations our young female students or young student wives had been subjected to. There was no demographic prevalence of any diseases in their country of birth. I concluded that there is a factor of abuse from the American doctors who knew that these students and their families were treated for free and any billing they submitted would be honoured and reimbursed for any procedure performed and even the length of stay in a medical institution is under no control or limitation. When it came to dentistry, huge bills were submitted for dental work on what was supposedly a healthy, young student population.

Working and planning closely with the statistical department and the marketing department of the health insurance company, we created a list of medical and dental procedures that were not reimbursed by the health insurance program unless a second opinion and in certain cases a third opinion, were obtained. So, a twenty-one-year-old female was not allowed to undergo a hysterectomy unless she obtained a second and a third opinion from different gynaecologists. This was mandatory to protect the female students and the wives of the students. I elected to pay for the consultations fees rather than the female losing her uterus because, for those countries, it was a cultural ignominy for a woman who cannot bear children. The same was applied for a list of procedures under the dental program.

To explain the new set of rules and procedures requiring second and third opinions, I circled the United States twice, visiting the students at the universities explaining how to utilize the health insurance program benefits and what were the effects and benefits of the second and third opinions which were initiated for their protection and welfare. I was available by phone during working hours for all inquiries in regards to the utilization of the health benefits. My success in developing the health insurance program after one year broke a record-saving four million US dollars. The health insurance program cost to the country dropped from nine million US dollars to three million in a year. This was welcomed at the home country with lots of praise to the administrators of the students studying abroad program. The safety measures were highly appreciated since it protected the students and their families from the American doctors seeking to perform unnecessary procedures. Although it was still a high cost, the foreign government used to allow students to come study in the US with family members who had complicated medical conditions ranging from psychological diseases to complicated untreatable forms of cancer. That was why the cost was high though only a handful of these cases were affecting the high health care cost.

The health insurance program was a success and my utilization profile analysis exposed the greed of the American doctors who were taking advantage of a lucid flow of money. I couldn't understand how a doctor would allow himself/herself to earn money doing unprofessional, unnecessary procedures for young foreign students who placed their trust in these doctors for their own and their families' lives. On top of that, in the end, I discovered that the ambassador of that country had a business relationship with the broker who used to administer the health insurance program before I took over and used to obtain a kick back from the money billed to the country through the health insurance program. What a shame, rich people put greed in preference to honesty in taking care of the young generation that was supposed to bring the country to a high level of social status and development when they got educated, returned to their homeland, and started working in the government.

Before leaving the student health insurance program administration, the success of the program triggered The Arabian Gulf Council to send two health undersecretaries from two countries to look into how to better offer health benefits to all Arabian Gulf students studying in America. Upon their arrival in America, I arranged for a health insurance conference with the top five health insurance companies in America. The health insurance companies' representatives answered all their queries and I prepared an idealistic health insurance program to offer socialised health insurance benefits to all the students from the Arabian Gulf countries under one umbrella of health coverage, under one health insurance plan and administered through one health insurance directory. The project was documented and sent to the Arabian Gulf Council and unfortunately stayed in paper only, since the countries could never agree to join hands and come together under one program. It was not clear why they didn't want to come together, maybe there were personal advantages from key organisers in each country to keep programs separate as we have experienced in the program I was administering.

CHAPTER 8

Exploring Alternatives to Dirty Medicine

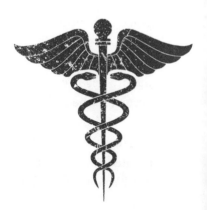

Frustrated, disgusted, depressed and saddened by the experience in America, I decided to return to my home country and start a private medical practice to exercise what I had learned by helping sick people. All dreams of specialization went up in smoke, so I would practice as a general practitioner and forget about specializing in surgery. My grandad had a big house in the centre of the capitol. I was welcomed to live with him since my grandma passed away and he was living alone. I refurbished the home to make it livable for him and my family. I built a walk-in clinic next to the house's entrance. I supervised all the construction and installed a water tank to have continuous water supply and an electric generator to have substitute electricity when blackouts occur, which was of common occurrence. The clinic was designed to handle general medical problems and at the same time had a small surgical room where I could perform minor surgical procedures under local anaesthetic. I had to bring all my medical supplies from overseas since what was needed couldn't be purchased from the local pharmacies. Being a new clinic, the influx of patients was very small, but I was happy practicing medicine with honor and honesty without the bias of any external influences.

Opportunities of dirt and greed passed my way, but I declined them, being in control of my own destiny. One of these incidences occurred when a Muslim girl wearing a hijab visited me in the clinic and asked me to perform an abortion on her since she was pregnant. I told her that I did not perform such procedures. She pointed to the picture of Jesus at the reception desk and asked me, "You are Christian, so what's to prevent you from doing an abortion? Besides, I can pay you thirty thousand pounds to perform the procedure."

That was a lot of money for an abortion; it was close to US$20,000.00. I asked her how she got pregnant. She said it was a mistake with her boyfriend. I told her, "As you fast and pray, I fast and pray too. It doesn't matter to God whether one is Christian or Muslim. I cannot perform an abortion unless it is a medical necessity. When I received my medical license, I took an oath that prevents me from doing abortions, besides I can't kill an innocent baby because you made a mistake. Mistakes can be corrected and you can let the person you slept with, approach your family and get married to you. This way, the problem is solved and you don't need to do something illegal both in front of the law of the land and against your religion. As her reply, she asked me if I knew anybody that could perform the abortion for her. I apologised to her and told her that I did not know anybody who would do it and I didn't want to know anybody who would have performed it.

There was a well-equipped private hospital which was non-operative. The doctor who started and owned the hospital was deeply indebted to another doctor. To get rid of the debt and the legal ramifications, he claimed mental incapacity and left the country. I researched the project and found out that the family still owned the premises and the furnishings with the equipment. I planned a project to make this hospital functional again. I approached the family and was given permission to invite different doctors so we could purchase the hospital from a medical group and form a group medical practice.

I prepared a business plan, had some of my friends as investors and circled the project to the professors in the different modalities that I had trained and worked with after qualification. I submitted the business plan and formulated the influx of patients having the health insurance experience from the time I administered the students' health insurance program in America. One of the largest proposed accounts was the worker's union where thousands of workers would have been covered by a health insurance plan through the services of the private hospital. All professors from the different modalities attended the invitation and we performed a thorough inventory of the hospital furniture and equipment. Everybody was impressed by the business plan. The next step was to finalize the offer and proceed with the purchase.

As is a usual occurrence in third world countries, a military coup took place and the democratic government was over-thrown and replaced by a military regime which started to crack down on all unions and private sectors. Of course, the military was anti-American, and I started to worry about my three children who were born in America and were American citizens. Next, the military government started to inforce Sharia law (the Muslim Law) on the people.

Tragically, the government hanged one of our fellow Christians. He was a co-pilot working on the local airline, and was charged with smuggling US dollars out of the country. His father was a priest and was negotiating a deal with the military personnel for a way to get his son released from prison until the trial date. However, the government hanged the son at ten p.m. without notice and handed the corpse to the family around eleven p.m. We were gathered at the family home when this happened. There was no time to react since there was a daily curfew from midnight to seven a.m. While gathering in front of the priest's house, I told all members of the community and those who dwelled at the suburbs of the city, that we would follow the curfew and would all meet at the church at nine a.m. The curfew was usually lifted at seven a.m.

Next morning, thousands of people gathered in the church, pouring from all suburbs of the city. I was talking to our archbishop about a plan that after the funeral ceremony, he should allow us to march with the coffin from the church to the cemetery. I requested the route to pass through the American Embassy, so they can record and document the incident as proof of the atrocities against Christians.

While discussing the route, a human rights activist from the American embassy and his assistant came to meet with us. He was the second secretary of the embassy. He asked me not to plan any violence during the march. I told him that we, the Christians, do not use violence and we do not even own or know how to use firearms. We were trying to document that, we the Christians are discriminated against and that this incident was a living proof of the military government actions against our people. Having the plan in place, we proceeded with the funeral prayers in the church.

When the funeral prayers were complete, the archbishop gave an order that nobody should march in church deacon clothes nor should anyone carry any crosses out of the church. I was carrying the coffin on the left front side. I was intentionally on that side so I could be able to direct the route of the march as was planned to pass in front of the American embassy.

Some uninformed people wanted to march in front of the presidential palace and chant slogans against the government. However, I succeeded in directing the coffin march according to plan by telling the other members carrying the coffin that we were taking the route in front of the American Embassy rather than the presidential palace and that this was permitted by the archbishop After peacefully and safely crossing through the first barricade of the military personnel who cocked their machine guns, ready to fire towards us, I lead the march all the way to the Christian cemetery. I did not use any anti-government slogans but chanted the first piece from the Divine Liturgy of St Basil the Great during the offerings of the bread and wine in preparation for Holy Communion during the Holy Mass, Kyrie Eleison which, when translated from the Coptic language means Lord Have Mercy. It is usually sung forty-one times in representation of the forty-one lashes our Lord and Saviour Jesus Christ was subjected to before crucifixion. The chants were:

Kyrie Eleison, Kyrie Eleison, Lord Have Mercy

Kyrie Eleison, Kyrie Eleison, Have Mercy upon us
O Lord

Kyrie Eleison, Kyrie Eleison, Hear Us and Have Mercy upon us

No anti-military slogans were allowed either, to avoid any clashes with the secret service and the military soldiers. They had orders to shoot.

We arrived safely in the cemetery and the coffin was buried. One of the Muslim locals was following the march and when the coffin was being lowered, he pick pocketed one of our people. He was caught and the person started beating the thief and wanted to bury him with the coffin. We detached them and prevented him from getting into trouble especially when the secret service personnel pulled their pistols to stop the beating. Thank God that incident ended safely and all participants returned to their homes mourning the lost member of the community.

The project I presented for the hospital establishment was on the table of the head of the worker's union when he was arrested protesting the military actions against the union. My appearance as a leader to the march, made me more vulnerable to be arrested especially when a Christian pharmacist was arrested and tortured. I took him to the American human rights activist's home. He showed the activist his lashed back with all the wounds. He told him that the military people made him crawl on the dirt and they were shooting around him. They were joking when he was frightened and told him that his education and social status meant nothing to them and he had to suffer because he was against the government and what they were doing to innocent people.

My fear for my safety and the safety of my family continually increased. I realised that there were some people watching the clinic. I placed a notice on my clinic door that I will be leaving for a week overseas and that the clinic will be closed. While I made arrangements to leave to a neighbouring country, I came to know that England, Germany, Australia and Canada were accepting refugees according to the Geneva Convention of 1945. I decided to leave the country seeking safety for myself and my family.

Since the kids were born in the United States, I decided to leave for Canada and claim refugee status, at the same time, I obtained entry visas to England and Germany from the British Embassy just in case we were not accepted in Canada. Before completing the week vacation I had advertised, I returned to my home country, found my wife had already prepared the kids and some of our belongings, and we flew out of the country to Toronto, Canada leaving everything behind.

I called our relatives in Canada from the airport since we hadn't had a chance to communicate with anybody before the success of our escape. We stayed with our relatives for a week then applied for refugee asylum in Canada. The Canadian government was very generous with us, started a refugee claim and they gave us money to rent an apartment and to buy food for the family. We were not allowed to work, for in the early nineties, the rules were restricting work only to Canadian residents. A lawyer was assigned to our case through legal aid and we waited for the refugee tribunal till our hearing.

I had given up on Medicine from the bad experiences I lived through for many years and especially since I had exhausted all my options. However, there was a group of female doctors in the church trying to sit for the qualifying examinations of the Canadian Medical Council that qualifies foreign medical graduates to be recognised for medical practice in Canada. They asked me to join them in the study group. Since I was not allowed to work and had nothing to lose till the refugee hearing was scheduled, I accepted their invitation and joined the group sharing my experiences with them.

They told me that the University of Toronto was issuing equivalency certificates for foreign medical graduates. The University of Toronto had an equivalency office for all foreign educated individuals. I contacted the office and applied with my certificates. They evaluated the Bachelor of Medicine and Bachelor of Surgery as equivalent to a Bachelor of Science from University of Toronto. We argued about the equivalency since the Bachelor of Science is a four-year course with basic science syllabus, while we had studied Medicine for six years and had the syllabus of medical schools. They were very rude and inconsiderate and they mentioned that this was only to help us find a job, if we didn't accept their evaluation, then they would issue nothing. Hence, we accepted the equivalency certification since we did not have any Canadian school certificate and might be useful in the future.

My friends at the church convinced me to study with them and to sit for the Canadian Medical Council qualifying examination. As refugees, we were allowed to enroll in classes and sit for exams without restriction. So we prepared for the examination, borrowed the exam fees and sat for the qualifying examination. After few months, the results were out and five of us passed the Canadian medical council examination. This proved that we were recognised as physicians whose education and training were acceptable to the Canadian Medical council. I applied to different hospitals and was contacted by four different hospitals in four different provinces. I was prepared to leave Ontario and go work anywhere. I had the belief that the Canadian Medical system would reignite the dreams and ambitions to accomplish my plans for my future in Medicine.

The local governments in the four different provinces refused to issue me a temporary license to practice medicine in spite of the hospitals' need and acceptance to enroll me within their staff. One local government gave the excuse that while I was in America, I did not practice medicine for two years and I was working in Health Insurance which was not medical practice. Although the hospital and I both argued that I had returned to medical practice after that period, they still refused to accept the plea. They required that I had to pass Part 1 of the licensure examination of the Canadian Medical Council. So, I got stuck again in rules and regulations that didn't make any sense. The hospitals needed my skills and the local governments refused us entry into the Canadian Medical system.

Determined to pursue our careers, we started preparing for the Part 1 licensure examination. The examination fee was CD$3000.00 and the exam was three days duration with 900 medical questions. That was a brutal exam, even some Canadian medical graduates found it very difficult for we sat for the exam at the University of Toronto with their medical graduates. When the results were issued, I scored sixty-five while the required pass mark was seventy-five. That was the time that I gave up completely on medicine.

It just wasn't worth it—I had three kids to take care of. So, I started researching didactic programs close to medicine to try enrolling in them, get a certificate and when settled, I could find a job to feed my family. I looked into the different options in front of me. I found out that I could study and qualify as a medical radiation technologist. The modality was related to medicine and patient care, and I could earn a reasonable income and with my wife's education in business administration, we could earn a decent income to feed our kids and settle in Canada.

In my research and during a visit to the open house of the health sciences institute, I found out that Nuclear Medicine is a challenging program that requires two years of didactic studies followed by one year of hospital training. X-ray and radiation therapy were other programs for consideration, but the nuclear field was more interesting. I applied for the Nuclear Medicine program which had the modern applications of radiation to diagnose disease and was a highly computerised specialty which would be very exciting and challenging to learn especially coming from a third world country that had no computer applications in the practice of medicine.

The results of the admission process came out, they were looking to enroll forty-five students; I was not one of them. Since applicants had the right to investigate why they were not accepted through the registration process, I called the registrar to find out what happened. I was told that the candidates who applied had a higher qualification than me and I was high in the waiting list in case one of the accepted students declined admission. So, there is nothing to do, I had to wait and see how this would turn out.

I one day suddenly received a phone call from the institute and was informed that if I wanted to enroll in the program's academic year, I had to bring CD$2000.00 within two days and come to register at the institute. I was able to arrange the money thanks to my relatives and went to register.

I had to take the bus from where I lived to the train to go to downtown, connected with the TTC subway to a station close to the institute and then walked to the institute. I didn't mind that since there seemed to be light at the end of the tunnel for an opportunity which would allow me to obtain a specialty qualification in Canada that helped diagnose sick people. For me, diagnosing a disease using technology that would allow sick people to receive the correct treatment was as good as treating the patients from their disease.

During orientation, I was shocked to find out that four students in the program were right out of high school, another was a foreign male dentist, then there was me and an Indian female foreign medical graduate. The rest of the thirty-five enrolled students had different master's degrees from various Canadian universities.

The didactic program was very interesting: learning about radiation sciences, radioisotopes, chemistry, nuclear physics, patient care, and anatomy. Since I used to be an instructor in university teaching anatomy, the institute had a policy that any student can be exempted from the Anatomy class if he/she scores a grade of 85 or above. I challenged the exam and scored 94, so I was exempted from attending Anatomy classes and practical. I completely dedicated myself to my studies and to learning the technology, and as a result all my scores were averaged at 80. I was elected as the students' representative for the program sitting in on the nuclear medicine advisory council committee meetings. After two years of didactic studies and practical, I completed the requirement to be placed in a teaching hospital for clinical training.

The year of clinical training was divided into three-month intervals, training in different modalities of Nuclear Medicine. I completed the first six months by training in general Nuclear Medicine at a downtown general hospital and pediatric Nuclear Medicine in Sick Kids, the children's hospital. When it came to the radioimmunoassay shift, I completed the three months but the clinical director wrote a bad report on my performance. She never liked me and had showed a discriminative attitude towards me from the start. I neglected all her negative attitude for the sake of survival. That turned out to be a reason for the director of the Nuclear Medicine program to kick me out of the program. Are you kidding me? I couldn't just leave, especially after investing all that money and the effort of two and half years of hard work and study in a program that I liked and was scoring high grades.

One of my teachers liked me very much and was always supportive through the whole period I was studying and training. She advised me that I had to fight my case in front of the advisory panel. She further informed me that the director of the Nuclear Medicine program had the policy of admitting foreign medical graduates to the program and then finding a way to kick them out so she could say that the Nuclear Medicine program she was administering was of high standard and that foreign medical graduates who were qualified physicians in their home countries, could not complete the course because it was difficult for them. Over the years, there had been many foreign medical graduates accepted and then were subsequently kicked out of the program. In reality, there was no foreign medical graduate who completed the nuclear medicine course in the history of the institute. The instructor helped me to prepare for my defense.

I entered the meeting with the advisory panel which was formed of different heads of departments in the institute, the program director, and the clinical instructor who wrote the bad report. I presented my defense to the panel against whatever the clinical instructor had reported. The panel was astonished at what they heard; the only two in disagreement were the program director and the clinical instructor who wrote the report. The panel reversed my dismissal and instructed the program director to change the site where I completed the previous three months and instead report the result of repeating only a four-week reassessment cession in a different hospital.

To further make things difficult for me, the director placed me in a hospital in London, Ontario which was 160 Km away from where I lived. She could have placed me in a closer hospital, but she expected that I would decline the placement and that would be grounds for my dismissal from the program. I had to complete the reassessment period, so I borrowed additional money and left for London, Ontario.

I had a very old car so in not depriving the kids from my attention, I lived in a motel in London and used to drive home on Friday evenings after my work at the radioimmunoassay lab, stay with my family for the weekend, and late in the evening Sunday, returned to the motel. That was expensive for me, but to pursue my new career, I was determined to complete the assignment to prove to the panel that what I had presented in my defense was accurate.

I scored 100% in the four weeks assessment. That allowed me to return to my family and stay within the program to obtain my qualification. When I met with the program director, she told me that I did very well and scored 100% in London. I didn't reply to her remark.

To complete my clinical training in Nuclear Cardiology as a selective subspecialty, I was deployed to the downtown general hospital. The last three months were completed without incident, and I presented the required project to complete my clinical training.

On the last day of my clinical training, my assigned instructor who supervised my clinical work, placed me in a chair in her office and proceeded to say very bad things to me in an attempt to upset me into starting a fight. But, I kept my cool and accepted all the disgrace she poured on me for I understood this to be the institution's method of assessing their students, by stressing them out exceedingly and, if they tolerated the stress, then the instructor would sign off their passing grades. What a pathetic method of assessment.

Securing a Canadian qualification and registration with a Canadian Association, you would expect to have a job lined up to practice what you have learned. Unfortunately, in the mid-nineties, the job market was bad for medical radiation technologists and jobs in the field were scarce. So, after years of hard work and studies, I had a Canadian certificate and obtained a Canadian citizenship—but no available jobs.

There were, however, shortages of medical radiation technologists in Australia. Since there was a reciprocity agreement between the Canadian Medical Radiation Association and the Australian and New Zealand Medical Radiation Association, my qualifications would be recognised in Australia and I could work there as a Medical Radiation technologist in Nuclear Medicine. I arranged with relatives in Australia to go there with my family.

Arriving in Australia, after few months, I was able to secure a temporary part time job in a hospital far away from where I lived. I used to take the three a.m. bus to connect with the train downtown, and then take another bus to reach the hospital by seven a.m. In the afternoon, I commuted the same way back to home. I continued to do that for four months till they opened a job posting in the department for a senior technologist. The director of the program was an African specialist radiologist in Nuclear Medicine. She wanted me to have the job since they were introducing nuclear cardiology as a new modality in Australia and, because I had the Canadian experience and was helping them in the set up and construction of the protocols and adjusting the radiation doses for the cardiac nuclear stress studies, I was interviewed for the position. The director told me that I did very well in the interview, but the hospital hired a technologist that graduated from Australia and that personal connections played a large part in the hiring process. Again, dirt surfaced in the Australian hospital system.

Keeping my options open and looking for further employment in the field, I met a Japanese nuclear medicine radiologist who had a private clinic with an Australian radiologist who committed suicide in the clinic. His chief technologist discovered the corpse when she came to open the clinic one day and the shock caused her such distress and psychological problems that she couldn't work for some time. He was looking for somebody who had nuclear cardiology experience to work in her place in the clinic. After the interview, I was hired in the clinic. This caused me to move the family to live close to the clinic. The clinic had two locations, so I had to cover for both locations on rotational basis.

In the main clinic they had a triple head gamma camera and used Thallium as the isotope for cardiac studies since its half-life is longer than the common new radioisotopes used in Canada. They used to import the Thallium from Amsterdam. Every day the radioactive drug was delivered to the hospital from the airport and we passed by the hospital to pick the package and bring it to the clinic on our way to work.

There was an Australian nuclear medicine physician who used to come from Melbourne to the north coast for reporting once a week. He was not friendly and continually repeated that we foreigners came and took the jobs from the Australians. At one time, I told him that he should not keep repeating this for the Australians were not educated in the nuclear field and there were shortages of medical radiation technologists. People should appreciate the help and experience of others in diagnosing patients. Eventually, the staff member who was unable to work because of the suicide incident returned to work, they hired a new graduate and had a student trainee in the clinic. My job became redundant since they were overstaffed and I was let go.

Things were not going great for me since the Australian system was completely different from the Canadian system. In Canada, we had a high standard of patient care and followed the ALARA (as low as reasonably achievable) principle in injecting radiation into the patients. I discovered that here the technologists inject the patients with a higher radiation dose so that they can complete the scans fast and go home. They did not use radiation protection protocols to protect the staff or the patients. Simple basics like using gloves while handling radioactive doses did not exist. Most of the time, they did not use radioactive shielding for the injectable doses. There was nothing called quality control on equipment they used for producing images. When a problem was detected, they would call the manufacturer for help. There were no trouble shooting skills at any level. I realised that I was working in an unsafe environment with lower standards than what I had learned and practiced in Canada.

In addition to this, my three kids were enrolled in Australian schools and they were not happy missing their friends and the Canadian environment of education. In addition, my wife couldn't find a job to help out. I started looking at all these negativities and evaluated our future in Australia.

Living there I found out that eighty% of Australians were living on social assistance and the Australian kids did not really work hard for they expected to rely on the same assistance when they grew up. There was a dull, unhappy feeling with the people living there and of course most of the older generation were drinking alcohol all day long. In the area we were living and working in, there were a large number of people with mental disabilities of different ages seen using public transportation and in the market place.

On top of everything, life in Australia was different from what I experienced in North America. Thefts were rampant. In fact, if you left your home for few days, you could expect to come back and find it wiped of all furniture and appliances. It could even happen if you left your home for a long period of time during the day. There were lots of incidents of jealous people entering homes and destroying the furniture which in many cases were expensive leather materials.

The environment was worrisome with spiders all over the place. Spiders can reach huge sizes, and in the schools, they teach the kids how to protect themselves from poisonous ones. In some places there were cockroaches—like millions of them—an everyday battle. Some places have rats, poisonous frogs, and you name it kinds of annoying creatures that make leading a regular, clean life a challenge. I decided to return to Canada for the sake of my children because it would be a crime for me personally to be selfish and deprive them of the opportunities they would have growing up in Canada in comparison to in Australia. At least being Canadian, they will receive a quality education, secure a future, and live in the environment of their choice. Having a dual American/Canadian citizenship, they will belong to the free world and will have opportunities that can lead to a nice, safe life and, hopefully, they will not face the difficulties I encountered in finding a place for them to grow up. That experience made me create a slogan about Australia: "It isn't worth living on an island, even if it is a continent!"

So I decided to return to Canada. Packed our stuff, sold my car and furniture and headed back to Canada. Jobs were still scarce after a year's absence. To feed my family and try to repay my loans, I worked as a midnight cashier in a grocery store. What a disaster, with all the qualifications I had, I ended up working a minor job in a grocery store: cleaning floors, arranging shelves, and selling cigarettes and groceries. I was attacked on a midnight shift by two thieves who entered the store with large farm knives and masked faces. They threatened me and stole cigarettes and the money in the till. When they left, I called 911 and reported the robbery, I called the owner of the store, and he told me to call the police and to tell them that the thieves stole lots of cigarettes and money so the insurance would repay him the damages. I told him, I already called the cops, and that he had no sympathy or compassion towards me; if the thieves killed me was he going to bring up my kids? The police caught the robbers because while I was on the phone they dispatched the description I provided to all police patrol cars in the area. Strange how people think only about themselves and feed their greed; the owner didn't care if the thieves killed me or hurt me and if I followed what he said to do, I would have been considered a liar to the police. I quit from the grocery store right away after the robbery.

 I found a job in two gas stations as an attendant. I started with the night shift and gradually walked my way to the morning shift in one of them and the evening shift in the other. At the same time, I worked in car detailing since one of the stations was considered to be one of the busiest car wash stations in Canada and the owner had the insight to add extra revenue by introducing detailing to his business operations.

 Still pursuing the Nuclear Medicine carer, I found a casual part time job in a hospital 180 km from where I lived. I used to hit the highway at four in the morning to reach the hospital at 7 a.m. to start the day. Sometimes, I had to work two to three days shifts so I used to sleep on the stretcher in the department and shower at the surgical suite showers in the surgery theater. I couldn't afford staying in a motel or hotel, the cost of gas was high, consuming a large part of my daily wage. I left working in the station for I couldn't get the days off when I was called at the hospital. I worked as a security officer in one Security Company which plans shifts in different buildings and had a flexible schedule. That worked out well since I could go work in the hospital every time they needed help and just skip the security duty.

At last, by the grace of God, I got a break! Through my job applications, I came across a radiologist who owned multiple private X-ray clinics with nuclear medicine and bone densitometry. He interviewed me and asked me if I was able to start a private nuclear medicine clinic at one of his sites. I showed him my skills and that we could develop a nuclear cardiology site since the modality was new to private diagnostic imaging in Canada. That was a big, challenging project and an opportunity to set up a diagnostic nuclear medicine environment that had all the basics of what I studied and laid down the foundation of a career and an attempt to make a name for myself in the diagnostic imaging arena.

I was handed a nuclear medicine license and a large room in a medical building. The X-ray, the bone densitometry, and the ultrasound were across the hall. I was expected to design and equip the room to create a new private nuclear medicine modality in the medical building. I designed the room in such a way that any technologist could walk in and function in the setup. The way I did this was by practicing radiation safety procedures for the staff and the patients, right from the door inwards.

I created a work station area where studies could be analysed, an exercise area with a stress treadmill, a change room for the patients to change their clothes and a nuclear laboratory with proper radiation protection shielding to meet the CNSC (Canadian Nuclear Safety Commission) standards. Working closely with the nuclear camera vendors, I installed the first double headed gamma camera of the millennium in a private medical imaging setup.

The patients would be booked through the X-ray department reception and I planned my working day so that the patients were injected with the radioactivity early in the morning, the day started at seven a.m., and rescheduled their return for imaging, timing their return so that the radioactive patient would not be waiting with the other patients in the X-ray department waiting room, for besides exposing the staff and the other patients to radiation, there were lots of pregnant ladies there for the ultrasound. For studies in nuclear medicine, the patient was injected with radioactive material and then left for a period of three to four hours drinking lots of fluids and going to the bathroom to clear the excess radioactivity and to give a chance for the radiopharmaceutical to concentrate in the area of interest for imaging. Cardiac nuclear medicine is performed in two settings, a stress portion and a resting portion, and then the images of the two settings are compared to detect any defects in the cardiac muscle. Depending on the radiopharmaceutical, the cardiac nuclear test can be performed with stress first, then rest or rest then stress and then images are compared.

The owner arranged for a cardiologist to supervise the stress portion of the cardiac studies. An internist sometimes used to come supervise the stress test. By law, the stress test can be performed with a technologist, but a physician has to be in attendance just in case something goes wrong, so the patient is not at risk. I used to prepare the patients for stress test and the supervisor conducted the stress test and at peak exercise, I would inject the patient with the radioactive tracer. I followed the ALARA (As Low As Reasonably Achievable) principle in ordering the radioactive unit doses and always maintained a low radioactivity dose that facilitated good quality diagnostic images.

Due to the striking success of the facility, the owner asked me to evaluate and expand his two other nuclear medicine sites. While performing my duties in the new clinic, I used to visit the other sites and prepare a scheme to upgrade and equip the sites to bring them to the latest level of nuclear medicine imaging.

At one site I found that they were imaging patients with a twenty-year-old gamma camera, the first generation of gamma cameras that was producing poor quality images. The other site had two gamma cameras, one very old and another that could perform cardiology scans, but was out of date. None of the sites had a patient stress environment. The owner hired an internal designer to remodel the old clinic and I was assigned to supervise. Of course, the internal designer did not have any knowledge of the nuclear safety regulations, so I had to redesign the design to meet the CNSC standards and regulations to keep patients and other staff members safe from radiation.

I arranged for a steel company to come dismantle the old gamma camera and use its hard metal as scrap. Working closely with the gamma camera vendors, I installed the latest gamma camera available at that time and structured a nuclear laboratory for receiving isotopes. I designed a separate cardiac stress area within the department and multiple examination rooms with the plan of accommodating and attracting visiting physicians to practice in the facility. The department even accommodated a shower where the patients could elect to shower after going through the stress examination, if desired. I arranged for a technologist to work in the facility and an internist to supervise the cardiac stress.

It turned out to be the talk of town with the latest technologies in place and a pride within the medical imaging community. My presentation for the upgrade of the other old private clinic fell short of execution. The site was disorganised, but the doctor who was sending the patients for cardiac studies had a very close relationship with the working technologist and they didn't want to change the set up they had for it was convenient and comfortable for them. The exercise stress treadmill was in the doctor's office on the fourth floor while the gamma camera performing the images was in the second floor. When the doctor was stressing the patient, the technologist had to take the radioactive dose up two floors to initiate the study. The doctor was afraid that if the setup was changed, he would lose the influx of patients who used to come to him. The site was neither upgraded nor changed and my recommendations and ideas filed.

CHAPTER 9

The Dirt in Medical Imaging

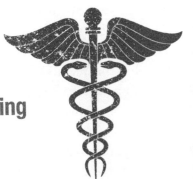

Jealousy from other technologists working in the different modalities at the private independent facility, started to creep in. Especially when one day they got hold of my pay stub. I had warned the owner not to send my pay stub to the clinic where I was working daily. I had sensed that the technologists who were working there for many years were not comfortable with the successes I had accomplished. They felt that the revenues I was generating and the reputation the clinic reached made them feel as if they were not doing enough to generate revenues all the years they had been working there. They started to gossip and make false accusations against me to make me look bad to the owner and since he had worked with them for years, he listened to them. Even employees in the company who were running the administration from another site, gossiped about my use of the privileges I was given, like credit card usage and travel allowances to the other sites.

 I worked so hard and proved that I could handle loads of patients per day working more than thirteen hours. I used to image twenty-five patients per day. In the cardiac nuclear stress studies, I reached a maximum number of twenty-seven patients a day working from seven a.m. till eleven p.m. There was a huge influx of patients from the doctors working in the medical building where our clinic was located. After some time, I came to know that this medical building was owned by the pharmacist who operated the pharmacy on the ground floor of the building. He and the owner of the diagnostic imaging modalities guaranteed rent free medical offices for all the doctors working in the building in exchange for prescriptions to the pharmacy and patients sent to the diagnostic imaging facility.

On top of that, the influx of cardiac patients came from one general practitioner who was known for his interest in cardiology and used to receive two cases of an expensive wine around Christmas time, each bottle costing CD$2,500.00. Around the holiday season, I found the owner upset and when I asked him about it, he told me that the doctor sending the cardiac patients called him and asked him why he hadn't sent him the customary wine gift he used to send every year. The owner told me that he sent him two cases of a cheaper but still pricy wine; he added that he had sent him the expensive wine on top of what he had sent already, and the doctor kept all four cases. So, the influx of patients was because of a dirty arrangement with the doctors who only care about receiving gratuity for sending the patients and having a rent-free office. The owner of the medical imaging focused his attention on the referring physicians in all the facilities he owned all around town in the different locations. He owned a medical building in town and he was doing the same thing with the doctors in the building.

I discovered that other independent, private health imaging facilities had the same sort of arrangement with practicing doctors, some extending their wicked dirty games at the ministry of health level and politicians to receive allowances not permitted in the Canadian system to other independent health facility (IHF) owners. All private imaging sites are under the ministry of health IHF program. The ministry of health disallowed licences for private independent health facilities since 1992 in spite of the growth in population.

In one incident, I was called by the referring physician who used to send the cardiac patients and he told me that the report he received for one of his patients could not be accurate since the signs and symptoms of the patient contradicted the cardiac report findings. I told him that could have been an error and I would check on the case. I double checked the report and reviewed it with the nuclear medicine advisor of the clinic who was an associate professor at the university. I found out that the professor of nuclear medicine in the university issued an incorrect report. The associate professor, who was our advisor, told me that the professor most of the time did not know how to diagnose cardiac studies for he had all his work in pediatric nuclear medicine imaging and that all cardiac nuclear studies should be sent to him and the other general nuclear medicine studies sent to the professor. Here, I stumbled on the fact that although the radiologist was not sure of the diagnosis, a report was generated just for the sake of reporting a study. If it was not for the alertness of the referring physician, who at least in that case had the good conscience not to give the patient medication on a suspected wrong report; I wouldn't have any suspicions about our cardiac reporting system. The professor and the associate professor with another female professor were the pioneers in radiology in the university and owned four independent health facilities performing different imaging modalities. It was sad to detect that some of the generated cardiac reports could be inaccurate. I intentionally avoided sending the professor any cardiac studies to prevent errors in treating the patients who trusted us. That was not the only incident, unfortunately I came across lots of reports which were incorrect and had to be reviewed to save patients from unnecessary treatment.

This, together with the staff jealousy and back stabbing, started to threaten my existence in my role as an advisor to the nuclear medicine operations. The owner reduced my pay without any reason and deprived me from the privilege of a private phone line I used to communicate procedures with the patients, the different vendors, and the other imaging sites, as well as the use of credit card and travel allowance. Hence, I resigned to explore other options.

During my research for other opportunities, I came across a nuclear medicine technologist who was running one of two nuclear medicine IHFs with very low patient volume and old equipment. With my reputation, I offered to help him. I advised him to relocate his practice and I would help him upgrade the equipment with my connections and set up a more modern facility. He had been abused with his partners and I gave him the idea to purchase his shares and own the license for the facility. I offered to work with him in case he elected to separate from his old partners. He accepted, and we actually moved his license to a facility which had ultrasound, bone densitometry, and an X-ray.

We offered the owner who was an ultrasound technologist a reasonable rent and added the nuclear medicine modality to his business. I set up the nuclear laboratory, the imaging area as well as a stress treadmill. We started our operations introducing nuclear cardiology imaging and the business was picking up. The owner of the ultrasound facility started to get greedy and he

The Dirt in Medical Imaging

wanted to collect extra money from the revenue we are generating. He was pressing the holder of the license to sell him the nuclear medicine license. He wanted to influence me to destroy the operation so he could purchase it and we work together. He missed one scenario: I do not do dirty business. I was honest with my fellow nuclear medicine technologist that I worked with and told him of the plans of the ultrasound owner. I told him that if the efforts to separate from his partners succeeded, I would partner with him and head to another location to restart. The frustration reached the stage that we had to move. At the same time, the other partners agreed to sell the license to the nuclear medicine technologist and we would have sole ownership. This was a trigger to look for another location and move the nuclear medicine operation.

For the third time, I created a beautiful nuclear cardiology clinic as well as general nuclear medicine imaging. I purchased a new double headed gamma camera and contracted with the internist who used to work with me in the first clinic whom I had helped a lot when he arrived in Canada and his private clinic was very close to our facility. He was our treadmill stress supervisor. We had another emergency room physician supervise some days depending on the influx of patients. We worked so hard and I managed the clinic and its revenue till all the equipment was paid off in a year's span. I retained the associate professor to report the nuclear cardiology studies since he was good and experienced and was one of the few who laid down the basics for nuclear cardiology. I trusted him. We had a couple of nuclear medicine radiologists who used to report for us, but I ended their affiliation with our operations since they were not up to the standards I laid out for the operations. Being a co-owner of an IHF, I had the ability to make decisive decisions and obtain and retain the best in the business. I was not going to be enslaved with the radiologist who believed that they can just report anything and without a care for the patients' welfare. I am the one who was doing all the work to generate good images and I deserved to have the best, honestly generated reports so patients can receive the correct treatment.

The operations were running smoothly and there was a massive influx of patients with huge revenue. Suddenly, my partner started coming to the clinic smelling of alcohol. In one incident, he injected a patient with the radiopharmaceutical ordered for another patient. I managed to scan the patient, for the radioactive dose was enough to obtain an image to diagnose his case; however, I had to cancel and reschedule the other patient. This happened twice. I told him to be careful to double check the scheduled patients and if he was in doubt, ask me or just let me perform the studies.

The one incident that made me mad, forcing me to ask him to leave the facility, was when he inserted a used butterfly needle in the forearm of a patient undergoing nuclear stress testing. He had no excuse to do this; I had tons of supplies at hands' reach. As a result, I told him that I could not work with him anymore in such an irresponsible behaviour and I wanted to end our partnership. Money and work are not everything in life, conscience and peace of mind is all that counts.

I didn't follow up on the patient; maybe he contracted Aids or hepatitis from that irresponsible action. I couldn't work in an environment that threatens patients' safety. I couldn't keep this partnership. I offered to buy him out, but we had a shot-gun clause in our agreement, so he gave me what I offered him, and I left the clinic and the partnership. I didn't report the wrong tracer injections, for those wouldn't have injured the patients.

But I couldn't let this serious incident go unreported. I reported the incident to the College of Medical Radiation Technologists. The college initiated an investigation. He brought two lawyers with him to the hearing trying to convince the panel that my claim was frivolous and that I was trying to strip him from the clinic. The college and the appeal board did nothing and they dismissed the case. I was disappointed that the College which was supposed to be there to protect patients did nothing in this case and I left him to his conscience.

I moved along to work in a general hospital in nuclear cardiology. Meanwhile, I was looking to purchase a nuclear medicine license. Nuclear medicine technology was dying out except for nuclear cardiology. Most of the scans that used to be imaged by nuclear medicine had been moved to MRI which uses magnetic resonance to obtain diagnostic imaging and prevents any radioactive complications from the radioisotopes used in nuclear imaging. This was a new modality that was worth exploring. While working in the hospital nuclear cardiology department, I started didactic studies online with the British Columbia Institute of Technology. In just over a year, I completed all courses and assignments and was ready to sit for the MRI examination of the Canadian Association of Medical Radiation technologists. To obtain a license to practice MRI I had to undergo training for 3 months in a hospital. To complete my clinical training in MRI, I requested 3 months leave without pay from the hospital to go join an MRI program to be able to secure my license. After completing my clinical training, I passed the examination and graduated with honors from the MRI program.

My stay at the hospital in nuclear cardiology was not without problems. Coming from private practice where I had control over the doses and used the ALARA principle, I found out that the hospital was using very high radiation doses to obtain images for cardiac studies. Furthermore, the reporting of the cardiac studies was done by cardiologists and not nuclear medicine radiologists. These were cardiologists who didn't have didactic training in nuclear radiology and had the ability to report nuclear cardiac studies by attending cessions of reporting from fellow radiologists. In private practice, the Royal College of Physicians and Surgeons banned cardiologist from reporting nuclear cardiac studies, while in the hospitals there were no rules governing reporting. In some places you find proper nuclear medicine radiologists reporting cardiac studies, in others you find cardiologists reporting nuclear cardiology images. The nuclear medicine technologists working there did the minimum work and were always fighting with me not to work harder for it would look like they had not been doing their job properly. In one occasion, they stopped me in the middle of the corridor and asked me to leave the patients and take a break. I refused and told them that I was there to work not to take breaks. After some time, I couldn't tolerate the toxic work environment and submitted my resignation. Now I had two imaging modality licenses, a Nuclear Medicine and an MRI, under my belt and I was qualified to practice them anywhere I liked depending on the opportunities.

An opportunity arose when I discovered a nuclear medicine IHF facilities business being liquidated. A nuclear medicine physician had a partnership that went sour when the partner was involved in a scandalous bankruptcy. They had to liquidate the assets of their two IHFs and their nuclear licenses were up for sale. I was interested to purchase one of the licenses since financially I could manage only one IHF facility and don't like to get involved in huge debts. After lots of meetings and discussions, I was able to purchase the nuclear medicine license, but it came with the condition that I had to give the nuclear medicine physician an advisory role with reporting privileges for five years. The license also included nuclear cardiology and bone densitometry. I declined purchasing the equipment in their facility since it was old and did not meet the standards of modern medical imaging. I prepared a business plan and submitted it to the banks. As a result, I was able to secure a CD$800,000.00 loan from one bank and a CD$250,000.00 from another. I still needed more than these million dollars to start the clinic though, so I had to borrow CD$300,000.00 from an independent lender.

I secured 1.35 million Canadian dollars to set up an independent health facility the way I wanted it to be without any outside influences or interference from any party. I would set up the clinic of my dreams the proper way with the precise rules and regulations IHFs were supposed to follow. With tons of experience in setting up diagnostic imaging clinics and having the knowledge of all the ins and outs of how things would function, I started searching for a location to the move the license to. Licences were allowed to move within a five km circumference in any catchment area.

I found a building owned by a cardiologist who was planning to set up a multilevel multimodality medical practice and dental office. That was a three-story building where on the middle floor there was a dental office. While in planning discussions with him, I suggested that the basement would be ideal for my clinic and the upper floors could be medical offices for different doctors that could utilize the nuclear medicine imaging. The building was very old and when I contacted my friend engineers and construction personnel, it was found that the building didn't have an adequately solid foundation to accommodate the heavy equipment of the nuclear operations. Renovations would cost the cardiologist lots of money that he didn't have for the building itself was an expensive purchase.

After few meetings, we didn't agree on a plan for renovations and I started looking for another suitable place. It was very hard to find a suitable location to start my clinic. After few months, I managed to find a medical building next to a subway station and a parking garage. The problem I faced here was that the available suite was on the second floor above the parking area of the building. After consulting with the nuclear camera vendor engineers, it was determined that the only way the floor will carry the equipment's weight was to reinforce the floor from above the parking space. Negotiating with the owner of the building, I offered a five-year lease under the condition that I would be allowed to reinforce the floor to carry the weight of the equipment. The owner agreed, we signed a lease agreement and renovations would start as soon as the floor is reinforced. It was winter time and the temperatures were sub-zero most of the time. I made arrangements with an engineering company that was experienced in reinforcing bridges. On contract, they had to create a warm net around the parking lot and installed heaters that were running for long hours to warm the air in the enclosed space, ensuring the roof would be warm enough to hold the carbon fibres they were placing in the area to be reinforced. In a week's time, the floor was reinforced and ready to tolerate the equipment weight.

I designed the suite in such a way that there were two interchanging change rooms in between the exercise stress area which besides the treadmill had a bed for intravenous pharmacological stress. There was a large scanning area where the double headed gamma camera would be installed and the processing computer station as well as the camera accessories. I designed three separate rooms for physician offices. An office for myself within which was a reporting radiologist station. A cardio-physiology room behind the reception where echocardiography with ultrasound equipment was available; in addition to blood pressure and holter monitoring. There was a bone densitometry room in the facility. The rented space was huge and during renovations, I hired a cabling company to wire phone and internet lines to all areas of the clinic.

The elevators in the building were small for transporting equipment. Therefore, the renovation team had to remove a window on the side of the building and widen the wall opening so that the machinery experts could crane the camera console and the imaging bed through the opening. That was a hectic operation but with good planning, delivery of the equipment was successful, and the renovation team patched the walls and reinstalled the window. Everything was done in the same day for it was January, and it was snowing.

At last the equipment was indoors and the vendor started the installation process. The treadmill and the bone density equipment were managed through the elevator and the safety stairway. Installation of all the equipment took approximately a month to complete. With the innovative new PACS (Picture Achieving System) gaining grounds in medical imaging, I installed a PACS system for enabling referring physicians to access their patient's images and reports once they had a log in ID. They were only able to access online the patients they referred and had no access to any other patients in the system to keep patient confidentiality to a maximum. The clinic was a beauty in the medical imaging arena. It was the first completely paperless digital imaging IHF facility in Ontario, Canada. It was equipped with state of the art equipment in medical imaging that used secure internet access by physicians, radiologists, and patients.

I had double and triple checked all the parameters of operations for a perfect execution. The CNSC (Canadian Nuclear Safety Commission) approved the nuclear laboratory as well as the patient waiting area, although they demanded very detailed nuclear physics calculations in relation to the radioactivity generated from the injected patients and the surrounding personnel.

The operations were ready to kick off in early March. I invited all physicians in and around the medical building as well as placed an advertisement in the local newspaper announcing the start of the new nuclear cardiology imaging facility. I contacted many cardiologists informing them of the new facility. The operations included general nuclear medicine studies, stress cardiac nuclear studies, bone densitometry, echocardiography, regular exercise physiology, blood pressure and holter monitoring.

The following was listed in the molecular Imaging website that belonged to the facility:

> *Founded by Dr. Nabil Basanti, Molecular Imaging is a diagnostic imaging facility which provides superior quality services to the community in Nuclear Cardiology, General Nuclear Medicine and Bone Densitometry.*
>
> *The wait time ideally is calculated from the onset of symptoms to treatment and rehabilitation. However in Cardiovascular medicine, there is no reliable method to identify the onset of symptoms from health records. Therefore, the measurable wait time begins at the point of first medical contact (visit to general practitioner or specialist, visit to an emergency room or a hospital admission)*

The Dirt in Medical Imaging

The Wait Times Alliance, a group of national specialty societies directly involved in those disciplines in which the first ministers of Canada committed to address the issue of lengthy wait times: heart surgery, cancer treatment, joint replacement, sight restoration and diagnostic imaging. They developed wait times for all of the provinces. The following are the Ontario times:

WAIT TIME ALLIANCE REPORT – ONTARIO

PROCEDURE	Urgent Wait Times (Working days)		Routine Wait Times (Working days)	
	MEAN	RANGE	MEAN	RANGE
Myocardial Perfusion:				
Exercise Stress	5	0 – 30	19	2 – 63
Pharmacologic	5	0 – 30	20	1 – 63
Bone Scan	3	0 – 10	11	1 – 30
Bone Density			29	1 – 150

MOLECULAR IMAGING SOLUTION

PROCEDURE	Wait Times (Working days)			
	EMERGENT	URGENT	SEMI-URGENT	NON-URGENT
Myocardial Perfusion:				
Exercise Stress	same day	1	2	3
Pharmacologic	same day	1	2	3
Bone Scan	same day	1	2	3
Bone Density			2	2

We have implemented those times to eliminate waits that are unfair, uncertain and that will create risks for the patients. While all involved medical parties with joint efforts with the Canadian Government are trying to reduce wait times, we dedicated our resources and finances to target facilitating a tremendous reduction in diagnostic imaging wait times in the three major deficiency areas as illustrated above. This was made possible by equipping our facility with state-of-the art diagnostic imaging equipment which facilitates speed in imaging together with superior, accurate and reliable quality diagnostic procedures. Our medical team work extended hours to accommodate our targets. Our PACS system enables our reporting physicians to report images through a secure web link. Our referring physicians can review the reports and images of their patients through a secure web-link. Continued on-going support and upgrades will be provided by the supplying vendors to ensure that our goals will be achieved as planned and established.

Our physicians and technologists credentials, qualifications and competence are approved by the Canadian Medical Council, The College of Physicians and Surgeons of Ontario, The College of Medical Radiation Technologists of Ontario and the Canadian Association of Medical Radiation Technologists. Our support staff is highly competent and qualified to conduct their duties. Our nuclear medicine physician consultant has been reporting studies for over 13 years. Our certified technologists earn continuing education credits on an on-going basis by attending seminars, workshops, and conferences in the fields of nuclear cardiology, general nuclear medicine and bone density.

Molecular imaging is labeled as the facility for the future, since our equipment is capable of future advanced applications such as PET and Hawkey SPECT/CT. Our staff is capable to operate and perform MRI images. Upon approvals for such services by the government of Ontario, we can implement these services to serve our community in a very short time frame.

OUR MISSION:

Serve the community through compassionate patient care and quality diagnostic nuclear

Cardiology, Cardiophysiology, general nuclear medicine and bone densitometry

OUR DIFFERENCE:

Superior Service and Patient-Focused Care

The nuclear radiologist I purchased the license from was the reporting cardiologist and the nuclear advisor of the facility. Lots of patients were referred to be followed by the bone densitometry equipment for follow up studies were needed to compare past results. For stress supervision I had an emergency room physician who was able to supervise the stress studies but declined reporting them. I didn't know why. But I sent all stress studies to a cardiologist through the internet to report the stress studies, blood pressure and holter studies. The emergency room physician and the cardiologist billed for their fees and I billed for the technical fees of the service. I had an assistant who was a foreign medical graduate from Argentina who had her training in exercise physiology during the same time I was working in nuclear cardiology at the hospital. I had all services covered by professionals to start the operations. The influx of patients began and I literally, personally visited all the physicians in the Toronto area, close to and distant from the clinic explaining what benefits they would obtain by referring their patients to us. For example, reporting was delivered within two days after completion of any examination. There was no waiting time for any service provided since time management, accuracy, efficiency, and superior patient care were the goals of my operations.

The first day we performed thirteen cardiac rest and stress patients. I had an emergency room physician who supervised the stress tests and a cardiologist to report the results. This emergency room physician was not comfortable reporting the stress test results but was comfortable supervising the stress tests. He was paid his supervision fees while the reporting fees were paid to the cardiologist who was reporting the holter monitors, the blood pressure monitors, and the echocardiograms. I was able to perform echo on cardiac patients by having a sonographer bringing his portable echo equipment to perform echocardiography on cardiac patients. This presented a complete cardiac workout for the referred patients so their physicians would have a complete picture and make an informed decision on the patients' treatment.

When the reporting nuclear physician reported the cases, she indicated that six of the scanned patients required cardiac catheterisation for she detected cardiac lesions on the imaged patients. I usually review all reports before releasing them to the referring physicians and cardiologists. I was amazed, shocked, and disappointed in the findings she reported. I had stressed the patients on the treadmill and performed their nuclear images, and my expertise in the nuclear cardiology field showed me that there was nothing wrong with the heart studies of these patients. What that nuclear medicine radiologist observed were either breast attenuation on the scanned female patients or a diaphragmatic attenuation on the men scanned.

I called her and told her my opinion on the reported scans. She was offended and told me that she had twenty-five years experience in nuclear medicine and that the reports were correct. She double checked them on her computer terminal at home, the one I supplied her for speedy reporting and indicated that the reports are correct and I had to release the reports to meet the forty-eight-hour reporting deadline we were committed to. I had no choice but to release the reports to the referring cardiologists. The response was bad! One of them asked me to send the reports for a second opinion; another told me that he would no longer send any patients for the inaccuracy of the reports. I consulted with the associate professor who used to report my scans for years. He confirmed that the six reports I sent him were wrong; he re-reported them correctly and I sent them to the cardiologist calling him and offering my apologies.

I didn't want to document anything on paper to avoid any problems at a later date. I told the reporting nuclear medicine radiologist who was my nuclear advisor and from whom I had bought the license and committed to a five-year contract, that she would no longer be able to report the cardiac cases, and that I would hire another nuclear radiologist to report the cardiac patients; she would have all the other nuclear scans to report. She refused and told me that her contract was without any exclusions and she would mandate to exercise her right to do so. She did not admit to her error and I realised that the only mistake I did in the whole operation is that I didn't check on the validity of her reporting and her reputation. I did not suspect that a chief nuclear medicine radiologist working for twenty-five years in a reputable hospital nuclear medicine department would release cardiac reports that were wrong. I was left with a scenario that I had a very well set up nuclear clinic with state of the art equipment, a PACS system for sharing images, with superior patient care and excellent imaging skills, but unfortunately with unreliable reporting.

I consulted with the associate professor who was an advisor for the royal college of physicians and surgeons; he informed me that to prove that the reports were wrong, all the patients had to undergo cardiac catheterisation and if it is proved that there were no lesions, then there is a case against the reporting radiologist. He indicated that it would be an impossibility to be approved by the college of physicians and surgeons to prove wrong doing by one of their members, and the patients might not accept going through the catheterisation. I had to tackle the situation on hand wisely. I was on the edge of bankruptcy since I had to pay the interest on the loans I had from the banks and the private loaners and the influx of cardiac patients had stopped from the radiologists. At the same time, I was working part time in MRI in two different hospitals to maintain my skills and flourish my MRI training.

I sought legal advice of the situation. The lawyers informed me that the only way to get out of the contract with the nuclear radiologist was to sell the clinic. Meanwhile, I was facing a lawsuit from a general practitioner with whom I was in negotiation to be an investor in the project since he had lots of money and showed interest in the project. During the initial preparations and planning, he was not involved, but was advised that he would be a partner if he shared in the start-up costs. During the negotiations, he started to play games and avoided direct involvement, so I decided to cut him off. In spite of the fact that he hadn't participated in any way with the set up, and we had no written agreements, he raised a lawsuit expecting to collect millions for being promised to be a partner and was cut off the original discussions. So, I had another problem that would hinder the sale of the clinic. During that period, the associate professor and his partners sold out their four nuclear clinics to a company from Montreal. I found out roughly how much they sold the clinics for, so I put a price on my clinic and posted it for sale. Different people and doctors were trying to purchase the clinic. When I approached cardiologists I knew, all declined interest in buying. One cardiologist already had two nuclear clinics and showed interest to purchase. He forwarded a CD$30,000.00 deposit as a virtue of willingness to purchase. He contacted other cardiologists whom I already contacted in search of a partner. I was shocked to know that he was contacting cardiologists around me to form a group to purchase the license and the clinic.

    The cardiologist who used to report for me, visited the clinic for the first time when he knew that there was an opportunity to be part of a cardiologist's group to own the clinic. He was aware of the operations and was collecting revenue from reporting, yet never come to visit me. The cardiologist that was negotiating with me to purchase the clinic had a plan to involve five or six other cardiologists to form a group and had each pay a sum of money to come up with the clinic purchase price and he only contributed a small portion, if any. When I found out his plan to purchase, I called him and told him that if he didn't bring the money I wanted, there would be no deal with him. He asked for three weeks to finalise the deal. I told him I was not going to wait for him to try to find investors and I didn't give him any additional time. It was straight forward, if he was interested in the clinic, he could pay the amount I wanted and find investors at his leisure. He was not happy and told me that I was difficult to do business with. I told him I do clean, straight business and do not play games; if he was ready, bring the money and close the deal.

I declined any additional discussions with him and instructed my lawyer to return his deposit. This cardiologist had his wife running his other two clinics and a nuclear technologist administering and executing the business. I used to cover for them at times when the cardiologist started the business in the second clinic. He used to travel to the US to earn more income on a weekly basis. I found out that they abused the system by performing unnecessary bone scans on their patients who were known to have chest pains due to their cardiac disease. The patients used to ask me why a nuclear bone scan was performed on them while the cardiologist knew that the chest pains were from their heart. Although I agreed with them, I couldn't tell them that they were exposed to unnecessary radiation for a bone scan so that the business would make additional revenue. My decision was to be harsh and straight forward for I knew from past history how they operate their business and I didn't have time to entertain them.

Another cardiologist offered me an amount far below what I was asking. He presented a written offer through his lawyer. He did not negotiate and I found it an insult to just throw an offer without considering any compromise. He thought if he low-balled me, I would considerably reduce what I was asking. I declined his offer. Another nuclear medicine cardiologist and a cardiology group visited me and they were trying to have the clinic for a free ride. I declined all their offers and kept trying to sell the clinic.

I had a certain amount in mind that was competitive with other clinic sales and mine was far more advanced than the other clinics sold in the marketplace. In my research for the sale, I called a company that was new to medical imaging and they were expanding their operations. I asked them if they were interested in purchasing the license. I got them interested and invited them to visit my clinic. They were very much impressed with the set up and operations, for they had never seen a facility like this in the private clinics arena. The company needed to have a nuclear medicine modality in their operations for history showed that one of their managers sold the nuclear medicine clinics they used to own for no good reason.

After few weeks of negotiations with their lawyers, they agreed to purchase the clinic in spite of the lawsuit it carried. Thanks to God, working with lawyers from my side and theirs, they purchased the clinic with a hundred thousand dollars less than the asking price. They pressed me to accept a CD$100,000.00 less than the asking price to cover the left over debt of the equipment. I wanted to be free from all the hassle that was going on around me and so, I accepted.

I continued to defend the lawsuit with the general practitioner. That took close to a year and in the end it was settled out of court. It cost me CD$85,000.00 in lawyer fees and the settlement was CD$55,000.00. It was so stupid of him; if he had asked me for that sum of money, I would have given it to him instead of letting me go through the aggravation of the lawsuit. He had to pay his lawyer too, very pathetic and unprofessional. I came to know that all the money that private practitioner had was through scamming people: working with the lawyer, he sues them and settles out of court, what a way of living, this was supposed to be a doctor who treats patients and has sympathy towards people. This was an example of how dirty medicine was practiced in the profession.

To quote one incident from the same general practitioner: one time he referred a patient for a bone scan. The patient was complaining of pains in her bones. I performed the scan and when the report came back it showed multiple lesions all over the body indicating cancer metastasis. We requested the X-rays performed on her, it showed multiple fractures on multiple ribs where the patient was complaining of pain. There were some on the arms too. The associate professor told me that the radiologist who reported the X-rays missed all these fractures since the report with the X-rays showed no abnormality detected. I came to know that the general practitioner had an X-ray technologist from oversees who used to be a physician and he reported the X-rays he performed. What a misery, to collect professional fees from the government and not to care enough to have a licensed radiologist to report X-rays, and risk exposing the patients to disasters. This was a sin that God would not forgive in dirty medicine.

After everything was settled, I began to pursue my MRI specialty that I received with honors at the age of fifty-two. Searching all around the country, I found a job in Nova Scotia at a district hospital North East of Halifax. The hospital had MRI equipment with no technologist to perform any scans. They used to have part timers from the surrounding districts come occasionally to perform MRI scans. I negotiated with the director of medical imaging and was invited for a visit and interview and to check out the facility. I showed him that I could create an MRI department for the hospital and design the latest MRI protocols practiced around the world. I was a member of the International Society of Magnetic Resonance in Medicine. I visited and had educational training at the GE Health Institute in Milwaukee, US two times. I had the expertise to write the protocols, lay down the safety procedures and create an MRI department. I was offered a senior technologist position and in few weeks collected my belongings and flew to Nova Scotia. I shipped my car through a transport company and my personal belongings with Federal Express. I stayed in a motel arranged by the hospital for three weeks till I found a place to stay. Houses and condos around the hospital were not up to the standard I expected, and it was difficult to find accommodation. The hospital through their real estate agent found for me an apartment which was part of a hotel complex. It was furnished by hotel furniture and was clean and acceptable. I rented it and received my car shipment and belongings there. It was only a few kilometers from the hospital.

The challenge was that I was given an idle 1.5 Tesla MRI magnet, there were no protocols written, an automatic intravenous injector, had all the coils for imaging with the exception of a neurovascular coil that images the brain and cervical spine in one setting. I started operating the equipment and writing the protocols as I was scanning. I started by creating a basic protocol for each of the body systems. There were three radiologists, two of whom had MRI training; the third had minimal exposure when he was doing his radiology residence. I wrote the protocols for all required studies. Every time I applied a new protocol, I got approval from the radiologists before applying it to the patients. I dictated safety procedures and taught the receptionist assigned to me how to follow what was required for patients' safety. Screening was done over the phone but I screened all patients coming to the department, explained all procedures to be performed and made sure that they were fit and safe to undergo an MRI examination. I obtained their signed consent and proceed with the examination.

I had my time very well organised and the hospital brought to me a student to train before he went to another hospital for his clinical training. I helped him a lot and trained him with the basics for proceeding to his clinical training.

Not all connected with the MRI department were so well organized however. In fact, many who worked there lacked time management and the cardiologists were not as efficient in their duties as they could be. They wanted to report from eight a.m. to four p.m. then go home to their families. They didn't care about the wait time. And that wait time on the MRI waiting list was massive: it was several months before a patient could get an MRI scan. I, however, organised all studies, prioritising all sick and needy patients and within about six months, I had gotten the wait time for the MRI requests under control. The technologists from the other imaging modalities were telling me not to scan more than eight patients a day. I don't know who initiated this rule, but on several occasions, to have a wait-time free department, I scanned twenty-five patients a day on a seven a.m. to four p.m. shift.

You might think that those in the MRI department would be please with this efficiency; but, no! The radiologists intentionally started delaying my working pace by showing up late. One of them used to go hunting before coming to the hospital, others would leave early to go curling. They started requesting scans for minor fatty swellings that could be diagnosed by ultrasound. One of them seemed interested in my proposal to establish a private MRI practice focused on performing only extremity MRI studies

The Dirt in Medical Imaging

and freeing-up the large hospital magnets for complicated MRI studies. They did not want to get involved in the innovative new MRI protocols however.

In one incident, neurologists from the city requested a cerebrospinal fluid (CSF) flow study. They asked me if I could perform the study. I told them to forward a protocol, and I would be able to perform the study. They put me in contact with the senior technologist where the study was performed. After some discussions and obtaining some parameters, I was able to write a protocol for the study since they had different equipment manufacturer. When the patient was referred, I injected the patient with the MRI contrast agent and performed the CSF flow study. It was beautiful to see the CSF flowing through the brain ventricles. When I presented the findings, the radiologist called me and told me that he didn't know how to report it. I told him that he should call the radiologist in the hospital where the scan was routinely performed and ask him how to report the findings and what to look for in the images. He declined to do so and, resultingly, wrote a report that was unsatisfactory to the neurologist who subsequently called me requesting the original MRI scan so that his own radiologist at the hospital could show him the findings. As far as I am concerned technically the scan was a beauty and showed all that he was looking for. I managed to send the scan to him and never heard from them again, though he used to send patients to me to perform the CSF flow study.

In another incident, when the Italian doctor in Italy discovered that there was widening in the internal jugular veins of multiple sclerosis (MS) patients and he was researching to determine if correction of the widening would make patients symptom free; next day after the news broke, the radiologists sent patients to my department. The radiologist in the department asked me if

I can perform the study to prove what that Italian doctor was hypothesising. I told them that I would research it and perform it on any patient referred. One of them told me that even if I discovered that the MS patients had a widening of the jugular veins, the surgeons in the province will not operate on them. My response was that our job in medical imaging is to provide an accurate diagnosis and then it was up to the patient to decide what he/she wants to do with it. I would not prejudge that surgeons would do nothing about a positive finding and deprive the patients of a treatment option.

I researched how to perform a flow study to show if there was any abnormality in the jugular system. I connected with all the MRI technological specialists whom I had worked with and had known through conferences. After trial and error, I wrote a protocol and was ready for execution. To be able to perform the study, I had to have a neurovascular coil that scans the upper chest, neck and the brain. Theoretically, if I could catch the bolus of my injection travelling through the arterial system to the brain then returning through the venous system to the heart, I could detect any defects in the blood supply system. While I was in an MRI conference in Halifax, I met a senior technologist in another district who informed me that they had purchased the new coil and, at that time, it would scan the whole spine and the brain in one setting and that they had a neurovascular coil that was sitting idle at their department. I asked her if I could obtain it by asking our manager to officially request it from their manager, for that would enable me to execute the new protocol I had written and try help the MS patients.

I succeeded in obtaining the neurovascular coil through our manager requesting it from the other district. The Italian doctor was right. Twenty-three patients out of the twenty-five patients

I scanned had widening of the jugular vein on one side. Of course, we were very popular after presenting the findings to the neurologists. Unfortunately, in Nova Scotia there was a huge prevalence of MS where no one had conducted any research to find its cause. Everybody blames genetics, but from my point of view, if the genes are coming from the Irish, then why is there no high prevalence of MS in Ireland? I personally suspect something to do with the environment and the food people are eating in the province.

The radiologists had started to resent my operations. They wanted me to scan only a few patients per day although we had a two day waiting period—Our district was the only one in the province to have a two day wait time for MRI scans—and patients from other districts were flowing into our department as a result. Patients didn't mind the commute from other districts if it meant they could have their scans performed in a timely fashion, for the other districts had long wait times.

I prepared and presented a self-evaluation and comparative study between our district and the other six districts in Nova Scotia. It showed that our district was the best at performing MRI studies and utilising the facility to its maximum. I even discovered that the radiologists were charging the province CD$700.00 for reporting MRI knee scans. They threatened me to not bring this to the attention of the management. Things were getting bad and they were causing a significant annoyance to my work and without any basis. In addition to slowing me down, they were pushing the receptionist to not book patients and attempting to reduce the workload. So, instead of being grateful that their department had the best performance in the province, they wanted to slow things down.

The MRI student had by now returned to our department after completing his clinical training. They pressured the student, now a registered technologist, to give them all details about my operations and used to take him curling to find out if he could function without me there. I trained him honestly and very well and equipped him with all what was required to operate the department. When they were sure that he could run the department the way they wanted, they wrote a bad report against me to the chief executive officer so they could get rid of me. They succeeded in terminating my employment by using a new manager of medical imaging who was hired from Saudi Arabia and the department was without a manger for more than three months. They played their dirty games and I left the hospital. Through the union, it was determined that it was wrongful dismissal and we settled at arbitration with a small amount of money since I only worked there for two years and the lawyers advised me that even if I took the hospital to court, I wouldn't get a big compensation. I returned to Ontario and formed my own advisory service offering my expertise in Nuclear Medicine and MRI for a fee.

While I was in Nova Scotia, I presented my Extremity MRI project to the minister of health to help reduce the MRI wait time across the province. The minister of health through ministry personnel advised me officially in a letter as a response to my project:

> *"Your concern regarding the potential for the diversity of examination requests at Capital Health District Authority (CDHA) to negatively affect the wait time for MRIs (specific to the extremities) is noteworthy; however, introducing more equipment and (as your proposal*

indicates) a private option is but one solution. As a first step to address any existing MRI wait time concerns; including extremity MRI, an appropriate direction for the Department of Health would be to identify potential opportunities to better utilize the existing publicly accessible technology in our province. Rather than lack of equipment, this issue could be due to the underutilization of MRIs located throughout the province. Operational capacity may likely be a factor in current utilization rates. Nevertheless, further investigation is warranted."

In spite of this admission of incompetence, nothing was done to alleviate the problem of MRI wait times in the province.

In Ontario I reached out to many levels of government both federal and provincial. The federal ministry of health responded to my request for a meeting to present the project by not having time to listen to the solution of the MRI crises solution I have researched and ready to present. In the provincial side, I was in communication with the Ontario Health Technology Advisory committee (OHTCA) which is the body making recommendations to the minister of health and long term care about the use and distribution of health technologies in the province. Since they were application driven, I submitted my proposal and application which was unfortunately not welcomed and I was not given the chance or opportunity to present my project and solution to the MRI wait time crisis in Ontario.

This is the response I received from the OHTCA:

"Thank you for your interest in submitting an application to the Ontario Health Technology Advisory Committee

Dr. Nabil Basanti

(OHTAC) on Extremity MRI. OHTAC reviews the clinical evidence on health technologies and interventions. Your stated rationale for submitting to OHTAC is to develop the evidence base on the effect of Extremity MRI on wait times, not clinical outcomes. The technology you are proposing is merely a smaller MRI scanner and, unless there is something unique in how the scanner affects accuracy, it does not lend itself to an evidence-based analysis. As such OHTAC is not the right fit for your needs."

And so, roadblocks continued to prevent me from realizing my dreams for improved healthcare, to the benefit and betterment of all Canadians. It seems that the individuals in control of fixing the wait time problems are not interested to use the scientific approach towards any solutions. They are obsessed with the belief that the health system is performing well in spite of the wait time problems. They do not realize that the health system is aging and far away from utilizing any new ideas or innovative solutions to relief the agony of waiting patients and their right for readiness of diagnosing disease.

CHAPTER 10

My Family and Medicine

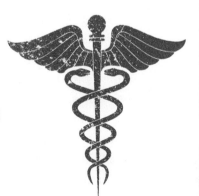

I had 24 year old twin boys and a 26 year old daughter when I returned to Toronto from Nova Scotia, Canada. One of the twins was complaining of pains on his right shoulder for nearly a year. Sometimes he complained of neck pains. After consulting with many doctors, he was referred to an orthopaedic surgeon at the hospital. After doing X-rays and some investigations, the orthopaedic surgeon began administering steroid injections to my son's shoulder. My son had to pay for the injections since it was not a covered procedure under the Ontario health insurance plan. When I started to look into his complaints and evaluating the history of what he was going through, new symptoms came into existence: numbness in the forearm and the thumb of his right forearm. I asked him to get an appointment with the orthopaedic surgeon and that I would accompany him to discuss these new symptoms.

We went to the appointment at the hospital. When we were called into the consultation room, we waited for some time and then the orthopaedic surgeon came to see us. He entered the room and didn't even greet me. He was told that I was the father. I heard what he was saying; he was suggesting proceeding with the steroid injections in the shoulder. I stopped him and told him that the pain and numbness my son was experiencing could not be coming from the shoulder. This was referred pain either coming from the brachial plexus (the network of nerves at the armpit that supply the forearm) or from the origin of the nerves at the side of the neck. I suggested exploring to find out if either was the origin; we should have an MRI for my son detecting the neck and the brachial plexus. He refused in the beginning and upon further discussing the case, he asked me why I didn't just write the requisition myself since I was a doctor. I told him I was not practicing medicine but I was a senior MRI technologist but could not request an MRI examination which would definitely settle this dilemma. He angrily wrote a request for a cervical MRI.

We did not get the steroid injection and after few months my son went for the MRI scan. While he was there, he called me asking me if it was okay for them to inject him with a substance and to obtain additional scans. At that moment, I knew that there was something majorly wrong. I encouraged him to proceed with the contrast injection and advised him to obtain the images on a CD. When I saw the images and the results came back, he had a tumour inside the spinal column pressing on the spinal cord. My suspicions were right that whatever symptoms he was experiencing in his neck, shoulder, forearm and thumb were coming from the compressed spinal cord pulling on the nerve roots exiting the spinal cord. I did not meet the orthopaedic surgeon again but he referred my son to a neurosurgeon in the same hospital.

Working in the field of diagnostic imaging, I detected that the tumour was five cm by three cm, extending from the second to the fifth cervical vertebrae. It had taken the contrast injected, so that means it has blood supply and was pressing on the spinal cord squishing it very narrowly at the tumor site. There were no swellings on top or below the compressed spinal cord and there were no widenings of the spinal canal. These were good signs as far as I was concerned, but what was the tumour: benign or malignant? Of course when you are in the medical profession and something like this happens, you go crazy subconsciously. I started researching the problem by going to the university medical library where I studied and trained. I researched all the scientific papers written for such a tumour. I photocopied ninety-four research papers to have a thorough understanding of what surgical procedures are used as well as what were the typical outcomes of such tumors. I didn't have a definite diagnosis so I covered all possibilities of malignant and benign. I even extended my research to medical textbooks. I did my due diligence and equipped myself with thorough knowledge about the case to intelligently discuss it with any specialist or surgeon. Of course, I needed to find a neurosurgeon that was specialised in operating on spinal cord tumors.

I was researching all the different hospitals through the internet to find a neurosurgeon that could operate on my son. I connected with some neurosurgeons, some were retired, others were working overseas, and others suggested that there were neurosurgeons in Canada that could operate on my son. The neurologist, who was following the twins because they were diagnosed with mild Tourette's syndrome while they were young, suggested a neurosurgeon specialised in spinal surgery at the university hospital.

We went to the appointment with the neurosurgeon referred by the orthopaedic surgeon. During the interview, he told me that he had never seen a case like this in his life and that he only performs one or two minor spinal surgeries a year on small spinal cord tumours. I asked him to refer us to the university hospital neurosurgeon and gave him his name. He got upset and asked me if I didn't trust him. I told him that I didn't trust him to operate on my son since he didn't have enough experience with large tumours and he only operates once or twice a year. He wrote the referral and we left his clinic.

Next day we headed to the university hospital where they had the neuroscience division. I looked for the neurosurgeon secretary and on finding her, introduced myself as a foreign physician and a medical radiation technologist in the fields of nuclear medicine and MRI. I handed her the MRI CD and asked her to attach it to the referral. In few weeks, we got an appointment with the neurosurgeon. He was a very nice gentleman, well versed from the way he was talking and examining my son. He told me that he needed to operate as soon as possible. And he would like to have another MRI scan before the operation at the university hospital site and that we would meet again for consultation before the surgery. After a few weeks, another MRI scan was performed with contrast injection again and we went for consultation. My research showed me that the operation can either be performed with an anterior approach reaching the tumour from the front of the neck or a posterior approach reaching the tumour from the back of the neck. We discussed both approaches and the neurosurgeon told me that through his experience, he prefers to proceed with a posterior approach and in case he couldn't remove the whole tumour, then he would re-operate and go from the front to remove any leftover tissue. He convinced me that the posterior approach was the best place to start. I accepted and we explained everything to my son. We waited to have the operation date.

After two weeks, the operation was scheduled and we went to the hospital. On the operation day, we arrived at seven a.m. where they prepared my son for surgery. They took him to the theater for the operation and me, and my family waited for him in the waiting room. I had my Bible with me and while they were operating I was reciting the Psalms. The operation took eleven hours. In the afternoon, the neurosurgeon came to meet us and told me that he was able to remove the whole tumour. He removed the arches of four vertebrae to reach the tumour and on completion he placed two rods to support the cervical column. It was a benign tumour but strongly attached to the spinal cord coverings. He said it was a schwannoma (a spinal cord growth from the coverings of the cord that was a very slow growing tumour and non-invasive). The neurosurgeon told me that he consulted with three other neurosurgeons overseas for the four of them were the authority in spinal cord tumours in the world. He told me that the other surgeons did not encourage him to operate since this was the first case in the history of medicine that a twenty-four-year-old young man develops such a schwannoma three by five cm in the region of the second to fifth vertebrae. Usually, these tumours are found in females and a little bit lower down the spinal column, extending from the lower cervical to the upper thoracic region. He added that they were suggesting radiation therapy in place of the surgery. I thanked him for his courage and in my mind I believed that God almighty had performed a miracle using the neurosurgeon to operate on my son to clear the spinal cord compression. All relatives and friends all around the world were praying for the success of my son's operation and asking God for a cure. God accepted our prayers and cured my son. I stayed overnight with my son at the ICU and the next day he was referred to the surgical ward. After few days, he was transferred to a rehabilitation hospital. The recovery was lengthy and after six weeks in the rehabilitation hospital he was discharged home.

My second son, the twin brother, was experiencing extra heart beats. He was working on a large construction project which was not going as planned and he was under lots of stress. He was referred to a cardiologist who performed an exercise stress test and holter monitoring detecting the extra systoles. He referred us to the hospital cardiac unit. We went and met with two cardiologists, one of them suggested that my son had an extra focus in his heart that is causing the extra beats. He suggested catheterization and cautering the site which is initiating the extra beats. He told me that there was a risk he could accidentally cauterise the sinoatrial node (the node that triggers the heart beats) and my son might end up with an external sinoatrial node operated by a battery. I didn't agree with what he was suggesting. How can he be unsure to mistakenly cauterise the sinoatrial node? What was he thinking? Did he want to experiment on my son? I told him that he was not sure of himself and that I would not allow him to perform any procedure on my son. I told my son that if it is not absolutely necessary, he should not accept such invasive procedures. We left the hospital and we never went there again. My son continued on the alfa blockers they subscribed to him to slow his heart. After some time the construction project was completed and the stress relieved. My son continued for few months with the medication and then stopped it. He never experienced the extra systoles again.

My mother had a fractured left hip. It was strange for she was complaining of pain on the hip for some time, and her family physician never X-rayed her. One day, she was getting up from the chair and she felt severe pain and couldn't walk. My niece called the ambulance and they took her to the hospital. When they examined her and did an X-Ray, they found the fracture. She was 76 years old at the time, so I told my sister that the orthopedic surgeon should perform a hip replacement to cure the problem. Next day, we found out that the surgeon had done a pin and plate for the fracture. The basics of orthopedic surgery dictate that any individual above the age of sixty-five should have a hip replacement for the pin and plates don't work. I didn't know if that was ignorance from the surgeon or if it was laziness to perform the replacement. I suspect that he intentionally performed the pin and plate so he could operate again on her when it didn't, work. Of course the operation didn't succeed and after a month he had to do a replacement for the hip. What an agony to the family and to my mom. She had a very hard time recovering from the second surgery which had a complication after few weeks and she was admitted for the third time to hospital to drain an abscess, luckily the replaced hip was not affected and they didn't need to reoperation and change the prostheses. What a waste of resources, time, and agony to patients.

I had fallen victim to the carelessness and lack of conscience of the practicing doctors. I had high blood pressure and was on medication. I never had a fixed family physician, every time I find one; he practiced for some time and then disappeared. They keep moving from one clinic to another and they don't care if you would find them or not. Anyways, there was a new medical building next to my condo and they were accepting new patients, so I went there to try my luck for finding a good doctor. I met a lady doctor who had a British accent and she introduced herself as a new physician coming from Manchester England. I felt relaxed with her and agreed to have her as my family physician. She tried to change the blood pressure medication I was on for years (I had an ACE [Angiotensin Converting Enzyme] inhibitor); she said the type I am using is old fashioned and she would use a newer brand. The newer medicine was very expensive and after she gave me some samples, I told her I wouldn't use it since it was too pricy for me. She changed the ACE inhibitor to an ARB (Angiotensin Receptor Blocker). I bought the medication and started using it. I began experiencing headaches and lower neck pain until it reached a stage that I went to see her and when she checked the blood pressure, it was 110/103. She was scared and gave me a letter to present to the emergency physicians at the hospital if the headache didn't subside. She stopped the medication and returned me back on the medication I had been originally using. Believe it or not from the first tablet, the blood pressure fell to its regular 170/85 which is still high, based on the medical literature.

She tried other medications in addition to what I was taking. We tried three other medications that all gave me complications of headache and neck pain and some made me feel very week and my ankles swelled like crazy. Meanwhile, she referred me to a cardiologist who ran a cardiology department in a hospital. I went to see him, and the secretary told me that they had to do an ECG and an Echocardiography before he sees me. I accepted the procedures so I could see him and ask his opinion. When I saw him, he was a young fellow who had lots of certificates on the wall behind him. During the discussion, he suggested that I do a nuclear medicine stress test to detect if there was any blockage on my coronaries. He said that there lots of people who had blockages and didn't know about them, I told him I don't think I had any blockages. He was trying to convince me and told me that the high blood pressure might be from a blockage. Here, I had to reveal my identity and told him that this was wrong, the high blood pressure would not be due to a blockage, the reverse would be true. Then during the conversation, he asked me if I trusted him. I told him I didn't know him enough to have any trust. I was an authority in nuclear cardiology and there was no indication for a nuclear cardiac stress test. I added that I didn't trust that he can read the nuclear cardiac images since he is a cardiologist and not a nuclear medicine radiologist who read nuclear studies after being trained to do so. He asked me if I knew how to read them. I told him of course I used to generate nuclear cardiac studies for thousands of patients when I was practicing medical radiation technology. I left the clinic giving him the impression that I was going to perform the study in the hospital. When they called me for the appointment after two months I told them I didn't want to do the test. The story of this cardiologist was that he specialised in invasive cardiology and all the income he earned was mainly from getting patients to do nuclear cardiac studies whether they need it or not. He earned lots of money reporting the studies; how depressing to earn a living without caring for patient's needs.

The other appointment in the cardiac centre in downtown came in after three months. I went to the appointment, met a cardiologist who asked me some questions and suggested that I might have sleep apnea. I told him I didn't think so, since I don't snore and sleep on my side. He still wanted me to do the study and prescribed another type of medication. I started the medication and was supposed to see him in a month time till the sleep study was scheduled. Close to my appointment time, they called me from the hospital and told me that the cardiologist had an emergency and would not be available on the scheduled time and gave me another appointment a week later. A few days before the appointment time, they called me again and said that the cardiologist would not be available and they did not know when he would be coming again. I told them that this is unfair. Didn't he have anybody to cover for him? I need somebody to see me and try to control my high blood pressure. After five phone calls and talking to different people, I managed to get an appointment with a cardiologist in two weeks. I went and met a female cardiologist who impressed me by examining me and showed care for my case. I revealed to her that I was a physician in my country of birth and that I was a radiation technologist in Canada. She gave me a diuretic in addition to the medications I was taking. After using the first cardiologist medication for a month, I started to develop headaches and lower neck pains. I emailed her and told her that I believe that medication is the reason for the symptoms. She was nice to communicate with me through emails which showed care and concern. She put me in a different medication to try reducing the blood pressure. It worked but when she wanted to increase the dose, I developed symptoms again. So, she left the original dosage to check if it will affect reducing the blood pressure. She suggested making an appointment with a blood pressure specialist who is a friend and a colleague of hers. I accepted and would go see her. My blood pressure came down from what I was taking and time would tell.

    I thank God I was the advocate for both my sons, otherwise they would have fallen within the dirt of the medical practice. When my patients used to ask me about their diseases, I always advised them to go read about their disease in a medical textbook discuss their case with their doctor. Once the doctors know that the patients are knowledgeable about their disease, they pay attention and watch what they are doing. The internet is not a good reference for medical problems; it has lots of junk written by unprofessional people. The best resources are the medical textbooks. If people do not understand what is written there, they can consult the nonprofessional versions of medical references or consult with a medical professional.

My seventy-six-year-old uncle, living in Mississauga Ontario felt shortness of breath. His family, wife and daughter, took him to the doctor who asked him to immediately go to the hospital. He was admitted and was told that he had water in his lungs. He stayed in the hospital for three weeks where he started to feel better. He was told that the investigations they performed showed that one of his heart valves was narrowed and he had to be operated upon in another hospital.

When he told me that, I questioned which heart valve? He told me he didn't know. The doctors didn't tell him any details. All what he knew was that they had made arrangements for the surgery in another hospital a week after discharge. I told him there is no need to perform surgery that soon for a heart valve narrowing doesn't happen overnight. It needs years to build up and if it is not eighty to ninety percent narrow, he shouldn't accept any surgeries. I suggested to him to go to the cardiac center in downtown Toronto to have a second opinion. He told me that he had full trust of the doctors and he would accept anything they say and there was no need to seek another opinion. I tried to talk him out of his thoughts but he insisted on his opinion supported with his immediate family who trusted what the doctors said to them.

My brother was visiting from the United States to check on my mom. He asked my uncle about the surgery. He told him that the cardiac surgeon told him that he would use the best valve which is expensive, and the government doesn't like performing surgeries with it. My brother explained the surgery in layman's words from the knowledge of how cardiac surgery is performed. He told my uncle that they will saw the chest bone and open up the rib cage to reach the heart. My uncle got scared and worried with astonishment on how it would be done. It was obvious that the doctors didn't explain the procedure to him. My brother cooled him down by telling him that the procedure is simple and is done many times in North America.

After few weeks, he went to surgery. They made all the preliminary investigations preparing him for cardiac surgery to replace the valve. When I asked him again, he told me that the valve is the large valve in the heart, probably the tricuspid valve of the left ventricle. He walked to the hospital the day of the surgery. They operated on him and strange enough the nurses instructed his family to go home for it will take a long time for him to recover after surgery.

My sister felt that this was not right so she went to the hospital and called his daughter to catch up with her. While my uncle was in recovery, he was asking about his daughter and requesting help for he was feeling uneasy. He wanted to go to the washroom and was trying to get out of bed. The nurses gave him a morphine injection which resulted in his heart stopping and they said they used a defibrillator to restart the heart. Then they said his kidneys were failing and they had to do dialysis but they did not have a dialysis machine so they would had to send to the other hospital to get one. Then they said he has high fever. At the end my uncle passed away in the ICU.

What a misery! It seemed that the cardiac surgeon didn't explain anything to my uncle who blindly trusted him without asking any questions and gave him the permission to do whatever he felt was the right thing. Probably he performed the cardiac surgery without transferring the body to a heart lung machine.

He experimented on my uncle and his experiment failed with my uncle dying. What a dirty way to practice. How can a doctor perform a surgery without explaining what he will be doing to the patient? How can they send his family away till he recovers from anesthesia? They all did what they wanted to do with neither passion nor good conscience nor empathy for the patient. If the patient doesn't make it, Oh well, he is a statistic. I came to know that there are lots of patients dying during valve transplant surgery in that hospital. It seems that neither this hospital nor the cardiac surgeon should be allowed to perform cardiac operations.

This should be a lesson to my readers that anybody who becomes sick should do his/her due diligence and discuss anything the doctors say to them and research it before allowing doctors to perform any procedure, so they don't end up as statistics. God forgive my uncle's sins and keep him with the angels in heaven.

My eighty-two year old mom was complaining of swelling on her feet and difficulty breathing. My sister took her to the family physician that after examination sent her for an echocardiography. Next day my sister realized that our mom's breathing was worse and told her that they have to go to the hospital and not wait for the echocardiography test which was scheduled in seven days. She was admitted as a heart failure patient in emergency next to their house in Richmond Hill, Ontario.

They called me and told me that mom was admitted to the hospital. I went there and found my mom in the emergency suite with an intravenous running. She was conscious and alert and was told that they are running Lasix, a diuretic, to help reduce the feet swelling and make her breathing better by clearing the lungs of any fluids. She stayed three weeks in the hospital getting better every day. The swelling subsided, the breathing returned to normal and she was planned for discharge. The cardiologist, who was supervising her care as an inpatient, told her that he is too busy in his practice and could not follow-up with her and that she has to look for another cardiologist.

What a pity! The family physician missed the heart failure! The cardiologist didn't have the courtesy to follow up on a patient whom he diagnosed and followed up as an inpatient. This is dirty medicine! I told my mom not to worry. I know good cardiologists in downtown Toronto in the Cardiac Centre where my high blood pressure was controlled.

I contacted the heart failure specialist I knew. She told me that she was on maternity leave but could arrange for her cardiology substitute to see my mom. She is one of the good doctors I came across in my career; one would be lucky to fall under her care if a cardiac problem arose. The substitute cardiologist saw my mom, she got registered in the Cardiac Centre and we were rolling towards the follow up in three weeks. He gave her some medications to help her because, on discharge from the hospital in Richmond Hill, the cardiologist just sent her home with a diuretic. My mom developed some complications from the medication. On contacting the cardiologist he changed the medication and then she was doing fine.

On the second appointment, the heart failure specialist had returned from the maternity leave and examined my mom. She planned her follow up and in few weeks saw her again to do some blood work. My mom's feet were swollen again but were of no concern. Of course, the heart failure has no treatment, only follow up and reduction of any edema in the feet and clearing of any lung congestion. I read the echocardiogram she had on the first admission. It was bad and depressive. She had atrial fibrillation, enlarged ventricles and mitral valve regurgitation. I was depressed for a long time since I knew she could pass away any moment and nobody can do anything about it. I kept it to myself and neither informed my brother nor my sister or any family member. It was hard to prepare for the unexpected all alone.

When my uncle passed away, my mom was very sad about his loss. We always sat and chatted about his case for neither me nor her could accept his choice to give himself to the mercy of doctors without asking any questions about what he had and what is the outcome of the treatment he would receive. Before the next scheduled appointment, which was in two months' time, the cardiologist emailed me and asked me to bring my mom to the clinic for her creatinine was high and asked me to stop one of the medications. When we went to the heart failure clinic, the cardiologist fellow told us that we needed to admit my mom to the hospital for the edema is too much on the feet and in the lungs and they needed to drain the fluids so she would have a better quality of life. She presented at that time with severe lower limb edema and shortness of breath upon walking, sometimes at rest and on turning in bed. They started an intravenous Lasix in the preparation room and in a couple of hours was admitted in the short stay inpatient cardiac unit. They continued treating her with Lasix intravenous injections. After a week they said she would need a continuous Lasix infusion and transferred her to an inpatient cardiac unit for long stay. They said that the nurses in the short stay unit could not follow continuous intravenous infusions.

In the long stay cardiac unit they hooked up a continuous intravenous monitor with Lasix. The maximum dose was given to try to drain the fluid from the lungs and feet. The lugs cleared but my mom started to have ringing in her ears and difficulty swallowing, side effects of the diuretic Lasix. They changed the

Lasix to two medications in an attempt to drain the edema. They started with a low dose and then kept increasing it to the maximum. During her stay as an inpatient, they performed lots of tests. Beside the high creatinine, they found an M protein in the blood and high Calcium. I asked the cardiology team to consult with hematology, endocrinology and nephrology. The former two came right away while the nephrology came after few weeks since they believed that the nephrology is consulted only for etiology and since they suspected Amyloid, they didn't need to consult with them right away. Every time the team comes with a test result or needs an investigation, I go back home, research it in the medical references and the next day I am ready to ask questions. I used to stay with my mom every day from 7:30 a.m. till my sister comes from work at 4:00 p.m. to stay with her till 11:00 p.m.

Let's take a look at my mom's case from the different angles:

CARDIOLOGY:

I had a very interesting discussion with the cardiologist from the team. He said that they consulted an Amyloid specialist from Princess Margaret Cancer Center and they recommend an Iliac Crest biopsy. He said that their survival prognosis for my mom is six months. I told him I already know that the survival rate for her heart condition is thirty percent survival for one year. But I don't believe in this; when she will go, this is something that God decides.

I don't think she has Amyloid heart disease. That radiologist or cardiologist who suggested amyloid in the echocardiogram was proved wrong by the PPY-nuclear scan which was even below normal. I believe the hardening of her heart muscle is due to old age. Whatever it is, the priority is to get the fluids out and try to get her mobile again. I don't believe in life expectancy; we are not God—the six months could be a couple of years. I have seen patients where life expectations were three months and they lived five years. I have the feeling that she will just go suddenly; God give her an easy time. I discussed this the day before with another cardiologist who with the nurse practitioner was suggesting palliative care. I told them as long as the cardiology team is working and trying to stabilize her fluids and get the edema out and monitor her I didn't have a problem but I didn't want to involve palliative care where they manage the end of life; I didn't want them to move her to a lousy place. I saw this before in my career and definitely didn't want that for my mom. The new diuretic seemed to work a bit but I think they were overloading her and the urine excretion dropped yesterday. If it is not effective we could try something else. I know it is difficult to get the fluid out, but we are hopefully trying to reach a stabilizing medication.

HEMATOLOGY:

I had a long discussion with the hematology doctor. My mom's blood showed a high M protein which is Multiple Myeloma and he agreed with me that the bone biopsy showed a poor percentage in diagnosing amyloid. I suggested a subcutaneous abdominal fat biopsy and give it to a good histopathologist to determine if it is Amyloid or not. Even if the test is 40forty percent conclusive it would give those diagnosing her condition, a better idea of what is going on. The Princess Margaret expert gave her opinion from looking solely at the paper work; she should have visited the patient to make an advised opinion. As far as Multiple Myeloma goes, everybody should exhaust all their investigations from the blood and do electrophoresis for that high protein and do the other tests in the blood to determine MM.

My mom would not tolerate an Iliac Crest biopsy and even if they proved it, she is not a candidate for Chemotherapy because it would not help her heart. The hematologist told me even chemotherapy would not prolong the six months expected survival. We agreed that there is no need to do an Iliac Crest biopsy. He himself told me that he was not comfortable doing these procedures nor does he like doing them. We agreed to take an abdominal fat biopsy to check for amyloid. And if it is negative they have to forget about anything else. He told me that all the blood work indicates Multiple Myeloma but that is irrelevant at this stage for she won't tolerate chemotherapy. So would do the fat biopsy to check for Amyloid and I told him let a good pathologist look at it and not just stain the sample and write whatever.

ENDOCRINOLOGY:

For the high calcium they did a total body X-Ray to detect any bony lesions. Nobody does this in modern medicine. A nuclear bone scan would have been more appropriate with low radiation. Anyway it was negative, so she had no bone lesions. She was scheduled for a nuclear parathyroid scan. They found an enlarged upper right parathyroid gland. They are suspecting this is the reason for the high calcium. They are suggesting surgery which is not a good idea since literature indicates surgery recommendation for patients less than 50 years of age. She definitely won't tolerate an invasive procedure to reduce her calcium. She responded to medication which was a good sign, so no need for surgery, her heart won't tolerate anesthesia.

NEPHROLOGY:

The renal team came to examine my mom. The urologist was a very smart individual who told me she is experiencing acute renal failure. He did not agree with the Amyloid diagnosis since all tests were negative. She doesn't have cardiac Amyloid. Her high calcium was mainly due to a secondary reaction due to the renal failure. He believed that the diuretic dose is very high, and the renal tubules are getting exhausted from the diuretic; they should reduce it and hopefully the kidneys would resume normal function. He said his team will follow up with her and see the progression of the case. I thanked him and connected with the cardiology team to reduce the diuretic dose.

PALLIATIVE CARE:

The cardiac team suggested involvement of palliative treatment. This includes involving community services with their nursing support and physicians. I told the cardiologist my only concern was that by involving them she would be sent home and we lose the hospital care. He told me that we need to involve them, so they can get to know her and support her and will be ready in case she returns home. I told him I was looking for help in getting her to lose all the extra water in her body, getting her up and walking, getting her in good spirits before sending her home for I had seen this before. He told me that the cardiac team will for sure be with her all the way, and it's good to involve palliative care to make use of their resources. Their representative passed by introduced herself and we had a long discussion about my mom's case.

So we agreed that there would be no parathyroid surgery, no Iliac Crest biopsy, no possibility of chemotherapy, and to continue the efforts to find a suitable diuretic and to concentrate on making my mom walk and having good spirits with free edema in the feet. We would only do the fat biopsy to establish a diagnosis for the Amyloid obsession.

The fat biopsy was performed by a plastic surgeon in their in-hospital clinic. This is a very simple procedure that can be performed by the side of the bed. I suspected it is because they want to collect more money. We just went ahead with it to satisfy everybody.

My mom was experiencing difficulty in swallowing. We asked for a referral, so somebody had to come and check on her. After two days, I had to push the nurses to check on what was happening. One nurse contacted the speech pathologist who informed her that there was no referral ordered. She spoke with me and I explained the situation to her. The speech pathologist told me that she would pass by and make her assessment. She came and examined my mom and said that the only thing she could do is to schedule a swallow X-Ray procedure to see what is happening. It was scheduled for next day.

Next day when I came in the morning, my mom was complaining of pain in her tummy. They said a doctor came saw her at night and gave her nothing for the pain. I asked them who the doctor responsible for the ward was that day. They told me that all doctors are in their rounds and somebody will come when they are finished. I told them she can't wait; somebody has to see her immediately. After an hour a doctor came, she examined her and took me aside and was telling me that my mom will not make it out of the hospital. We could elect to resuscitate her or not to do anything. I told her that we have to do our best for her and if she goes, then it's the Lord's decision not ours. We have to perform what we can to help her. I told my sister what the doctor said, and my sister was very emotional. I told her not to cry in front of my mom. I knew, now, that she would not make it and hoped for the best. After an hour my mom asked us to move her onto her side. I helped my sister to move her onto her left side.

I was talking with one cardiologist on the corridor when my sister called me and asked me to check if our mom was breathing. I told her no she was not. I called the cardiologist and he asked for a stethoscope and if she is a DNR (Do not resuscitate). My sister yelled "she is not!" My mom developed Pulseless Electrical Activity (PEA), also known as electromechanical dissociation, which refers to cardiac arrest in which the electrocardiogram shows a heart rhythm that should produce a pulse but does not. They called Code Blue – code for resuscitating cardiac arrest. They sent everybody out of the room and the team came in. I was in the room while they started CPR and medications to get her back. They tried many rounds for twenty seven minutes with no response. The heart failure cardiologist was with us in the room and she asked me what they should do. I told her it is enough she will not come back. They stopped. I closed her eyes and asked them to remove the endotracheal tube. I told them there is no need for an autopsy for it will be good for nothing. I called my sister and nieces to come say farewell. We lost our mom, God forgive her sins, and keep her with the angels in heaven.

It is very sad to realize that all doctors from different modalities look to treat their findings. I was disappointed that there was no communication between doctors and they did not take the patient as a whole. They only concentrate on their specialty and do not think of the other body systems involved. I had to brain storm for them to involve different specialties so that we could find a solution for helping my mom. It is very sad that those specialists reach high standards in their field and forget the basics of medicine where the patient had to be treated as a unit. I hadn't practiced medicine for more than forty years, yet, I found myself acting as an advocate for my mom discussing all aspects of her disease with top notch specialists in all modalities. I knew where to research in the medical literature every time they come up with something or a finding. The care in the wards is run by nurse practitioners and not by qualified doctors. Is this part of the dirty medicine? I can say it's an absence of treating the patient as a whole unit.

CHAPTER 11

Medical Radiation Technologists (MRT)

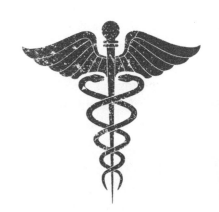

The following was published in the Ontario Association of Medical Radiation Technologists (OAMRT) Filter member's news magazine in late 2010 it was submitted without prejudice under the title of *MRT Identity-The Facts*. The OAMRT had a name change, now being known as OAMRS (Ontario Association of Medical Radiation Sciences)

I am submitting this article to be shared by all MRTs who are in the diagnostic imaging arena with the hope that it triggers an understanding of the facts about the MRTs' identity and will be fuel to the urge for MRTs to speak up and take the process of elevating their identity to be recognized by all stakeholders. Although this article mainly focuses on Ontario, it definitely reflects a pan-Canadian approach for I have visited, communicated and even worked for some time in other provinces.

I had been following the dilemma about the MRT identity for a very long time. I believe it was time to state the facts around MRT identity and to illustrate what brought about the muffling of the identity as it stands currently. I hope these facts will steer the directive of any organization or individual who will stand up and direct health care professionals, patients, all associations, government and the public to recognize the MRT.

The chair of the board and president of the OAMRT, in his message of the Filter edition of March/April 2010, presented a very interesting statistical review of the surveys conducted in this identity crisis. Did anybody read what the president wrote? In the July / August 2010 Filter edition, OAMRT rebranding task group recapped reasons why to rebrand. There was the CAMRT re-branding committee which was trying to come up with a new brand platform. It seemed there were two fronts trying to come up with a solution to the identity crisis. I do not agree with calling the process a brand (the first thing comes to mind was the use of the term in commerce as a trademark of a product or manufacturer or a product identifier). I would rather call it professional integrity. Both Filter issues and both messages talked about how the MRT was important in the health care system, how they were proud in performing their jobs, how good they were in treating patient needs, and how they were knowledgeable about the new technologies and their applications. No reasons given as to how the identity crisis came about and very weak solutions were provided poorly enforcing that the identity would be recognized only if the MRTs would introduce themselves as who they are.

Let's mention facts that everybody was avoiding – **THE TRUTH**:

THE RADIOLOGISTS:

MRTs fulfill the request of the radiologists in performing all scans either through coding of each requisition or a generalized agreed protocol in some modalities. The MRT has no input or say into what the radiologist dictates. **Here the MRT identity is muffled.** I would give an example: When patients were involved in a car accident, there were some radiologists forcing the MRT to perform X-Rays of all extremities even if there were no fractures or patient complaints. The MRT knows that this was not right, but cannot or would not say anything to keep it cool and to not disturb their relationship and jeopardize their employment. I consider this enslaving the MRT and accordingly MRTs would take whatever was thrown on them and this laid grounds for poor identity.

An argument might come that the MRT had not received the same training as a radiologist, but there were normal protocols acceptable to all DI modalities that the MRT was aware of through continuing education. MRTs know what was supposed to be done for the patient through knowledge and experience. In MRI, the radiologist will recall the patient to obtain additional income from a repeat study and would not make an effort to form a diagnosis using whatever images were already presented.

In Nuclear Cardiology, you find huge errors in reporting from radiologists who would report an inferior defect for a diaphragmatic defect and an anterior defect for a breast attenuation exposing patients to unnecessary cardiac catheterization. On the other hand, those cardiologists who think they were protecting themselves by enforcing nuclear cardiology scans to report on for extra income, exposed the patients to huge doses of radiation by scanning the heart with a double dose of radiation exposure both from Technetium, the nuclear traces, and the use of CT at the same time. There were lots of facts and examples that could be quoted in this regard. As long as there was no quality assurance or policing on how the radiologists or cardiologists were practicing and the hospital administrators were encouraging their attitudes, the MRTs would always be muffled, abused, and their expertise and point of view drastically ignored.

THE DI DEPARTMENT MANAGERS:

Most of the DI department managers were MRTs or technicians as they were called in the past. When individuals become managers, they forget their role as MRTs and get involved in the hospital administration bureaucracy and isolate themselves from the MRT environment. The DI managers who were technologists working in any department have passed through the radiologists muffling attitudes and enforce the radiologists attitude towards the MRTs so they can gain popularity among the radiologists and the hospital administration and thus secure their selection or job. **Here again the MRT identity is muffled.**

THE CHIEF/LEAD TECHNOLOGIST:

The chief/lead technologist was an icon of knowledge, power and execution. In past years, the **identity of the chief/lead technologist was muffled** towards following what was dictated by the DI manager, the radiologist, and the hospital administration. The chief/lead technologist was stripped from his expected duties enabling him or her to become a follower rather than a leader.

Medical Radiation Technologists (MRT)

To maintain peace and employment, he/she accepts whatever was thrown towards him or her enforcing it on other working staff and neglecting the rights of having input into any DI environment and thus a strong identity.

THE FELLOW MRTS:

Now let's look to the fellow MRT environment. Nobody stands-up for their rights or tries to improve the MRT environment. You see groups of people who aggregate with each other to have strength to be used to enforce their own wishes. Honesty, integrity, hard work, innovation, appreciation for others, were important identity resources missing from the MRT environment.

The MRT muffles his own identity. Wherever you go, you find groups of MRTs who were clinging to each other and would not accept newcomers, whether these were new graduates or other MRTs. If the new arriving MRT would not follow what the established MRT environment dictates, then he/she would be black listed and the MRTs start to cause problems or abuse the new comer till he/she leaves. If new comers accept what the group dictate, then he/she were all dandy and good another **self-inflicted muffled identity.** The new graduate faces the same crisis, and to gain work experience and to try to survive, hangs in there till he/she finds another employer. When they move from employer to employer, they find the same poor MRT environment and are faced with the fact that all working places have the same dilemma. Here the new graduate discovers the truth and faces the unfortunate fact that he/she just has to do the job. The ambitions and the willingness to improve the MRT environment were stifled and people sought employment survival, to at least pay the debt of their educational years. These facts were neglected, and the new graduates were blamed that they did not have the initiative to improve the MRT environment and most of them just do what was asked of them.

If you look deep into the MRT environment, you find fellow MRTs had a jealousy towards those MRTs who try to excel or be honest in performing their duties as MRTs. Any new protocol or procedure that was suggested always faced resistance. MRTs did not want to change what they were used to doing, even if the new suggestions would help them do their work faster and easier. MRTs did not accept change and always wanted to be told what to do. There was no drive towards progression and innovation. Very rarely you find a group of MRTs who wanted to improve but were powerless do anything beyond presenting their ideas to the radiologists and the administration. MRTs developed working policies of: "Do not do more than eight patients a shift"; "Do not work hard, they (hospital administration and radiologists) do not deserve it"; "If you work hard, administration would get used to it and you would make us look bad"; "If a patient canceled or did not show up, take a break, do not call another patient". These were actual working polices created by MRTs and were found across the board. As a result, **the MRT laid the grounds for muffling his/her own identity**. Of course human nature takes advantage of such actions and accordingly all involved parties in connection with the MRT enforced the deadening the MRT identity.

One fact about governing organizations, was that there was no communication between the different organizations. Each of them was a separate entity that tried to enforce certain rules and regulations to maintain a profile in front of the government and ministries or departments of health in the different provinces.

There are provinces that have their own regulatory bodies, that under the umbrella of self-regulation, enforced governmental regulations and assisted in muffling the MRT identity.

CAMRT (CANADIAN ASSOCIATION OF MEDICAL RADIATION TECHNOLOGISTS):

The CAMRT control MRT qualifications through conducting examinations. Registration with the CAMRT was a mandatory qualification for seeking employment in all Canadian provinces. It helped the MRT by providing a professional malpractice insurance coverage through the membership fees. This was the major benefit that the CAMRT was offering its members. When it came to continuing education, **CAMRT muffled MRT identity**—to qualify for another modality, the MRT had to go through the same courses that they had in their original qualification in addition to the specific modality to be able to qualify for sitting for an examination. That means the CAMRT does not respect the MRT qualifications and without consideration for the MRT's time and financial resources, enforces a set of mandatory course requirements to be completed prior to being eligible for taking a CAMRT examination. Why should MRTs repeat the cross-sectional anatomy, the physiology, and patient care courses that they had already passed through during their first qualification? This policy could be applied to foreign trained MRTs if their original course qualifications did not meet the Canadian standards. Fast crash courses for foreign MRTs offered by educational institutions were a poor measure of preparedness to face the Canadian MRT environment.

Depleting overseas MRTs from countries was not a solution to the MRT crisis that would hit Canada in the near future due to the aging technologists and the expected deficiencies in the workforce. The CAMRT had reciprocity agreements with some countries in the past. That helped MRTs and Canada to have ease of supply when demand in warranted. For whatever reason, that reciprocity was cancelled and instead of exploring new avenues in regenerating such helpful measures, the CAMRT elected not to bother for a reciprocity program and thus **locked the Canadian MRT identity**. In spite of the Pan-Canadian acceptance of the CAMRT qualification, MRTs in some provinces were forced to belong to the local provincial associations or colleges to meet the provincial requirement.

CMRTO (COLLEGE OF MEDICAL RADIATION TECHNOLOGISTS OF ONTARIO):

Under the umbrella of "protecting the public", the **CMRTO muffles the MRT identity**. The CMRTO focuses all its guns towards the MRT once a patient complaint had been initiated. The CMRTO navigates through different committees and procedures to investigate a patient's complaint. During the process, the CMRTO lacked the attention to detail and the MRT was perceived as guilty of whatever complaint till he/she was proved innocent, the reverse of our democratic legal system: "Innocent until proved guilty." The issues of sexual harassment, the obsession that MRTs may sexually abuse patients and the zero tolerance attitude, mandatory reporting, as well as the huge row around these issues enforced by the CMRTO, encourages complaints. The CMRTO does not have a method for identifying fictitious complaints; nor do they have a method for identifying patients who complain for the sake of obtaining a financial reimbursement, for that is an easy method of collecting easy money. The CMRTO do not appreciate the fact that in our current social environment and habits, individuals can have sexual relations away from the clinical environment. Female MRTs think they are immune from these sexual harassment issues, but within different social communities complaints had been reported from female patients against female MRTs as well as male patients against male MRTs.

In addition, the CMRTO failed to protect the patient from the extra tests that the patients were exposed to unnecessarily. There are lots of issues around this fact that the CMRTO neither has the expertise nor the resources to protect the patient. The CMRTO mission in protecting the patient has to go genuinely further than threatening, muffling, and controlling the MRT. In all the complaint cases in the history of the CMRTO, only odd cases had been proven to be true. This should not be a guideline to encourage patients to complain especially that the MRT community has no mercy on any MRT that goes through a complaint process even if he/she had been proved not guilty. The MRT is on their own if the complaints go to the legal system. The CMRTO has to appreciate the MRT and support him/her in any complaints rather than trying to justify the accusations.

When the odd case has been proven, you will find it in all CMRTO communications exposing the MRT's name and history; While when the MRT is found not guilty, the CMRTO doesn't have the courage to expose the not guilty verdict in their communications, **another MRT identity means of muffling**. The CMRTO has to bring pride to the profession by uplifting the MRT to have his/her identity appreciated by others.

The CMRTO strips the MRT from his title "medical radiation technologist" [which he/she earned from the CAMRT] if they are not registered with the organization. This title is a professional title that was honored to the MRT by passing the requirements set forth by the CAMRT to practice as an MRT. It is sad to know that most of the CMRTO staff were MRTs at one time of their careers. I presume that the other registering organizations in the provinces that have such colleges follow the same guidelines as Ontario.

OAMRT (ONTARIO ASSOCIATION OF MEDICAL RADIATION TECHNOLOGISTS):

It took seventy-five years of accomplishments and hard work from different members to bring the OAMRT to its current status. Unfortunately, the **OAMRT muffles the MRT identity** preventing them from participating with the other organizations. The OAMRT always refers and compares the MRTs to the registered nurses. There is an obsession with the nurses. The nurses are strong because they made their voice loud and clear. They can paralyze the health system when they go on strike, (a feature that the MRTs lack and can never achieve such a political tool in obtaining what is proper for them). Nurses scare the governments and they became so strong that they can do whatever they want in the system. When nurses were asking to write requisitions for MRTs to perform studies, the OAMRT got all hyper and everybody was excited about how a nurse could tell an MRT to do his work. Who cares, who writes the requisition. Much effort and time was wasted, and it still went through! Now when the nurses are performing an ultrasound, everybody is hyper and wants to fight it, so what? Doctors are doing ultrasound on the bedside. The OAMRT have to uplift the MRT identity and stop comparing the MRT with nurses.

If we develop our own strong identity, we can refuse an examination if it is not medically necessary. All MRTs and most of the senior technologists have enough experience to enforce this policy. If anybody does not agree, we are in the age of technology, a phone call to the radiologist or an email will correct the situation. The OAMRT being an educational institution, can enforce the radiologist assistant program, write the curriculum, develop the examination with the CAMRT and can force the radiologists to accept the change and those who qualify can control the MRT environment. The new scope of practice and expanded authorized acts that set a strong base for enhanced and advanced practice well recognized by government and other stakeholders does not mean anything for the MRT. The MRT can perform additional tasks that they were already performing through delegated acts without additional remuneration. So the radiologist and the hospital administration are benefiting while the MRT is overworked, **another OAMRT muffling of the MRT identity**. To uplift the MRT identity, OAMRT should have enforced an increase in pay for the MRTs (now OAMRS) by performing those new scopes of practice and worked to have MRTs control the environment.

MOHLTC – MINISTRY OF HEALTH AND LONG TERM CARE – ONTARIO

The MOHLTC has its own agenda and is still dictating to the CMRTO and the OAMRS in Ontario to follow what they dictate. The DI wait time crisis is an issue that the MOHLTC does not want to solve. There are lots of avenues and solutions that have been submitted to the ministry to lay the grounds for solutions for sick Canadians who do not deserve the agony of wait times in obtaining a diagnosis for their conditions and thus treatment. The MOHLTC **muffles the MRT identity** by not recognizing the MRT as the steering focus of the diagnostic imaging environment that they are enjoying. The fact is that they left MRTs to self-regulate themselves and as long as the regulatory bodies will muffle the MRTs then there will be no issues. Every now and then, the MOHLTC comes out with recognition for the MRT that gets all the different involved parties happy. It is unfortunate that those parties do not recognize the principals of politics that the MOHLTC successfully applied towards muffling the MRTs.

AHPDF – ALLIED HEALTH PROFESSIONAL FUND –

This was Health Force Ontario approach to make educational opportunities available to health professionals. MRTs were involved as part of the team. A political issue that aided in muffling **the MRT identity.** The fund was limited in its execution and not all MRTs were elegible to utilize it. It was not a matter of reimbursement; it was a matter of who were the MRTs that were given the opportunity to attend educational seminars or conferences to enhance their educational status. MRTs were not able to get time off from their working commitments to enhance their education. Some conferences encouraged members to attend a one day managerial wait time solutions presentation with a university professor who had no hands on imaging experience and based his educational materials on a purely business prospective. The cession cost the fund CD$900.00 per person, yet, attending the course resulted in no positive outcome to either the DI community or the MRTs. Looking to the fund idea, it was part of a political scheme to make everybody think that the government in Ontario was taking care of the MRTs practicing in the province. The fund only reimbursed the educational activity fees with no consideration to the attached costs to obtain the educational benefit.

PATIENTS

The CMRTO, OAMRS and the CAMRT have a strange understanding of the "patient". They all consider the patient as an ignorant, weak victim who is under the mercy of the MRT who is going to perform a diagnostic imaging test. All organizations do not want to admit that MRTs are dealing with highly educated, intelligent, computer savvy patients, many of whom know exactly what they will be going through. Many of the patients know **how muffled the MRTs are** in the system. In patient's observations, you can find the few who are appreciative of what the MRTs role is to those who would take advantage towards gaining monetary compensation by abusing the MRTs muffled identity. The fact is that most of the patients come through the diagnostic imaging departments demanding the procedures rather than listening to the MRTs who try to explain why they are performing the diagnostic imaging procedure. The fact is that the MRT is covering for the referring physician. Whether a consultant, or a general practitioner who doesn't have time so, falls short of explaining to the patients why they are requesting the tests. The MRTs are proud of how they handle patients, but unfortunately the odd cases against MRTs, enforces organizations to **muffle the MRT identity** and the MRTs are forced to consider the patients as a threat to their practice.

Now with the new requirements set out in the Health Professions Procedural Code of the RHPA obliging MRTs to have professional liability insurance, the MRTs working environment will be "hell in earth". Did any of the governing organizations realized that all CAMRT members carry professional liability? Why is the system burdening the MRT to take additional professional liability at his / her expense to satisfy a system? If the MRTs identity is not elevated to a superior level, all organizations will be faced with a huge deficit in MRT workforce for it is unhealthy to work in a threatened environment.

I hope I have tackled all the facts surrounding the MRT's identity and hope that by future years, individuals, MRTs, organizations or any party involved with MRTs will stand up and be courageous enough to fulfill their duty in advancing the professional integrity of MRTs.

The article had a good response from members and I received emails confirming the facts of what I had shared with the medical radiation technologists' community. Of course there were the odd technologists who resented the truth for they were practicing in a manner that is outlined in the article as to muffle fellow MRTs.

CHAPTER 12

Doctors Identity and Health Systems

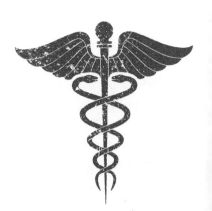

According to common understanding, a doctor is somebody who is supposed to be compassionate, kind and knowledgeable of how to treat sick people. In early times, barbers used to perform minor surgeries and people called them doctors. In the past people believed that there were some form of magical herbs treating disease that were given by some individuals and those were called doctors. Throughout history, the colonists and invaders of countries would experiment on local people with the medications they were creating to test the effectiveness in treating diseases. Those giving these medications were referred to as doctors. So doctors gained the reputation that they are knowledgeable of disease entities and were trusted that they have the means of treating sick people. This trust was passed from generation to generation and doctors gained the identity of being trusted in whatever they do and however they practice. Even in the current age of innovation and technology there are lots of people who blindly trust what doctors say or recommend.

Only a few people research their disease and discuss it with their doctors and if they are not convinced of the treatment methodology, they change doctors.

As we have explored in the earlier chapters, doctors are actually not what they were thought to be. In the British Empire, doctors were only from noble families. They were enrolling into medicine out of interest to offer healing to the sick and by no means as a source of income to better off their financial status. Those nobles had everything, so when they were practicing medicine, they were doing it to help the poor and sick. With the population explosion all over the world, there were not enough nobles to keep the tradition of wealthy people enrolling in medical practice.

Countries started creating medical schools linked to the basics of the medical education of the British. Medical schools started accepting students who scored high grades in the qualifying examinations for admissions in medicine. Interviews played a large part in detecting a student's fitness to enroll in medicine; of course, in many instances, students were accepted because they had a relative or a family friend in the medical field. The medical schools grew in number, and it became the norm that whoever scores high in grades, were admitted to medicine.

Education systems had its ups and downs, and through the years, each country has created their own rules and regulations for admitting students to medical schools, and after completing their didactic and training periods, to qualify for medical practice. Countries started to impose restrictions on accepting medical qualifications from each other and primarily accepted medical education if the medical schools were listed in the United Nations World Health Organisation registry of approved medical schools.

Huge numbers of doctors graduate from the medical schools and governments try to control their numbers by restricting medical school admissions, for doctors are among the highest paid in the working class. Most of medical schools around the world were influenced by British medicine. In North America, the medical schools gradually evaded the British system of medical education and the introduction of technology in diagnosing disease separated them from the traditional methodology of medical education, though all the creators of the new system were British educated.

The clinical sense training disappeared; now, doctors are trained on fancy medicine. They do not spend time following the progression of disease. They depend on technology to detect disease. Health insurance companies and governments force the system to discharge patients after a short hospital stay to save money. Doctors are paid fees for their patient visits and follow up. Surgeons are paid for the surgeries they perform. Obstetricians and gynaecologists are paid for deliveries and their treatment of female diseases. Radiologists are paid a fee for the number of scans they report. Family physicians are paid according to the number of patients they see per day. The labs are paid according to the tests they perform. Hospitals are paid for the services they perform. In Europe, the doctors are paid salaries from the governments. In America they are paid through health insurance systems. In Canada, capping of doctors' fees were introduced at one time, and as a result, you only find a few honest, good, and interested doctors who see their patients for free after their cap has been met, while the greedy take holidays after they reach their capped allowance. The colleges and the medical association succeeded in lifting the capping, but every elected government tries to bring it back.

For doctors to keep their financial status though, their colleges and associations influenced the government to lay down strict rules and regulations on foreign medical graduates who in order to enroll in the system of medical practice have to pass a series of medical examinations and licensure exams mainly created to deter enrollment into medical practice. Some foreign medical graduates break the system and pass the examinations and the licensure requirement, but where do they end up? Unfortunately, working the overnight shifts at hospitals and rarely given the opportunity to go up the scale like local medical graduates so most of them end in private practice. Immigration was influenced by local doctors and politicians restricted doctors' immigration with the excuse that there are too many doctors in the country. That through the years created shortages for doctors and there is now a huge deficit for doctor per capita ratio. If you are sick you end up in an emergency room that, in most of the hospitals, is run by a single doctor that cannot keep up with the influx of patients who end up waiting between six and eight hours to be examined.

When the government realised that the aging doctors are retiring, they started planning to increase medical school enrollments rather than looking into the vast majority of overseas qualified doctors who could save the system from the current crisis. So, the question arose: "Is it discrimination?" In the human rights code of ethics, education is not included in the list, though individuals are being discriminated against because they had their formal education in medicine.

Once people in the workforce know that the individual they are dealing with is a foreign trained medical doctor, they discriminate against him/her and do not treat them with fairness and freedom. You find lots of doctors working as taxi drivers or in gas stations to earn enough to support their families. It is not a matter that these doctors knew beforehand that they might not have a chance in medicine, it is a matter that these people have the right to come and live in the free world apart from whatever difficulty and discrimination they were exposed to in their home countries. The locally trained doctors are aware that those foreign medical graduates had a good education and training but fell short of the brutal unfair examinations they are required to pass and that most of them had high standards of medical education, ethics, honesty and superb eagerness to treat the sick, though some are the by-product of the policies of generating doctors.

Isn't that what a doctor is supposed to have in his/her identity? Unfortunately as we have read in the past chapters many American doctors were performing unnecessary surgeries on very young students studying in America because they could cheat and get paid without the control of a health insurance company. What about the 500 practicing surgeons in New York City who had never been in medical school? Most of the Caribbean medical schools have business agreements with hospitals in the US to take students for training. What a shame if American students who are good enough to pass the pre medical examinations qualifying them to enroll in American medical schools, yet, are passed over.

There is no short track in medical education; the student has to spend at least seven years within the medical environment to have a didactic, good, basic medical education and training. In Canada, you hear of a pathologist who was doing post mortems on victims of crime for more than twenty years and had sent lots of innocent people to life imprisonment for crimes they did not commit. When he was discovered and confronted, he admitted that he had not enough training. How could somebody not sure of what he was doing, present a report that affects the lives of families and testifies under oath to send innocent people to prison.

You hear of a radiologist who reports wrong scans and in the event of discovering the mistakes, it is too late for treating the patients and the patients die. Government forces colleges to investigate the cases reported and you don't know what or how many cases were wrongly reported and patients never know they had a wrong diagnosis. In my personal experience, I had the radiologist who worked for twenty-five years as a chief in a hospital department, reporting wrong cardiac scans I had performed in my clinic. How can the reports be signed and generated from a wild guess?

In Canada, the doctors protect each other for they have that analogy that if they are ever caught in a wrong diagnosis or something serious, the other fellow doctors will not testify against them, so they are safe within each other's protection. Contrary to America, when a doctor makes a mistake, he is slaughtered alive because of greed of other fellow doctors and lawyers. A doctor is paid a hefty amount of money to investigate and review a suspicious case of a mistake. When I was in America attending as an observer in a hospital, I came to know that the hospital is performing arthroscopies on any patient that came with a complaint of knee pain. When I asked why they were doing that? I was told that if any of the patients who is complaining of knee pain was treated and he/she ends up doing arthroscopy in another institution, and something was discovered, that there would be a couple of million dollars law suit against the hospital and doctor who did not perform the arthroscopy when the patient first presented.

When we used to break in the theater waiting room and the phone rings, some doctors would jump up in their seat, when I asked why, I was told that the phone call could be a million dollar lawsuit. So, American doctors are scared all the time, though they still try to fool the system and take advantage of any opportunity to make money. Greed, passion for richness, and carelessness defines the majority of a doctor's identity. There are good doctors out there but they are a minority. You as a patient depend on your luck. If you are lucky, you fall within the care of the few, if you are unlucky, probably you will be wrongly diagnosed and either it is discovered and you are treated or it is undiscovered and you die.

The college of physicians and surgeons are there to monitor the system and observe the doctors. They rarely admit to any wrong doing from doctors except in the very rare cases that the doctor screws-up big time and they cannot cover it. They know all that is happening, but they turn a blind eye, just to keep the system rolling. The problem with doctors' behaviours is that doctors can actually do whatever they want and there is no point in policing them. This is because the college of physicians and surgeons keeps the details of doctors' incompetence secret. In one example, details of a doctor's medical mistakes were kept secret from the public following a hearing that found the doctor guilty of malpractice with at least twenty-two patients. You can find lots of examples on the newspapers' websites. The same with the hospitals, there is no control on hospitals and they can do whatever they want with the money budgeted for them.

Health systems in North America are in big turmoil. President Obama was trying to furnish the poor Americans with a health insurance system that would help them to have coverage. When Obama-care was launched, the system had lots of glitches and somebody was trying to make the system fail. It launched and millions of Americans were able to have coverage. The system is good but needs some tweaking to perfection, at the most, people who never had coverage, would have one that could save their lives. Lots of patients benefited from this created system.

When Donald Trump was campaigning for presidency, he was against the system and he planned to revoke and replace it but without giving positive solutions. When Trump became president, he discovered that health systems are so complicated and all proposals from congress and the white house failed to dismantle a system that helps the poor get health coverage. The blame is put on health insurance companies, to their ignorance, health insurance companies are a processing organization that controls patient enrollments and pays the allowable fees for a service. One important issue is that the fee is decided on by doctors, so the origin of medical fees comes from what doctors' charge.

In Canada, the health system is so old and is nearly obsolete. Everybody from doctors to politicians is scared to introduce any changes to the system and always gives the reason that there is no fix to the problem. Canadians do not want to use technology to solve their health problems. They rely on economists to give them advice on medical issues. They avoid looking into solutions generated from within the system. I have researched and introduced a project for the governments to permit extremity MRI in a private setting and remove the extremity MRI scans from standard magnets at the hospitals. Forty percent of scans performed in magnets in hospitals are for extremity MRI. Those magnets should be free to perform useful studies that will help the sick and needy like detection of breast cancers and prostate cancers as well as detection of brain tumours. They have the technology, but the radiologists and administrators are resistant to apply it. The latter doesn't want to spend the money and the former is not humble enough to learn new diagnostic avenues. The Canadians brag about their health system in spite the all deficits and the huge cost they are acquiring to administer the system.

Lately in Toronto you find walk-in clinics on nearly each street corner. The doctors there work only a few hours a day and not a full week. In the hospitals, you find huge waiting lists in the emergency department because there is a doctor shortage. In third world countries, from where I am coming, the country was poor but it maintained the basic emergency room coverage in the different specialties. You find one or two house officers who are the first line of defense, then there is the medical officer and a registrar and on top the consultant. So each specialty has around five doctors covering it. You never find a waiting list. If Canada imposes this set up, the waiting time will definitely be eliminated. The government has to force doctors to work in hospitals and if they don't like it, they can find a job to serve their greed and laziness. I am not against doctors, but the fact is that they are the people who are supposed to serve the sick, not enjoying their lives by doing the minimum while being paid heftily in comparison to the rest of the population.

There are very good examples in Scandinavia and some European countries, so the Canadians need to be humble enough to seek advice from those countries where there are near-perfect medical practices. The Canadians have to utilize the modern medical technology in serving the sick, one of the very poor areas is that you don't find MRI centres for diagnosing breast cancer; all females are exposed to the mammography which is unfortunately read by incompetent radiologists. The literature has lots of examples that are unfortunately covered. Both federal and provincial health personnel have to be humble to seek solutions from individuals in the medical field and not from economists and non-health professionals. The system could be perfect but need a lot of work and courage to change and challenge those who resist.

The problem with doctors in the civilized world is that they are not humble enough to admit when they come across something they don't know, and won't ask another opinion. They believe that they would be seen as uninformed and incompetent. The other problem is greed; they want to make as much money as they can even by buying and selling patients. The ideal doctor who cares about patients and shows honesty and empathy is a rarity in civilised modern times.

I hope the reader is enthusiastically encouraged to research any medical problem he/she encounters in their life time. This is also extended to their family and friends. Reading through the incidents I have encountered and lived through, is proof of how individuals should cope with medical problems and doctors.

The ideal doctor, whom anybody can trust, no longer exists. Even the good doctor should be questioned and investigated when he/she is providing care. All individuals should research their medical problems in medical literature and not rely on the internet where most information is biased and inaccurate and in most cases is only the outcome of people's experiences.

I hope this book will encourage people to do their due diligence in handling disease and I hope they find the best doctor and care when they get sick, a reality that we all have to face at sometime within our life time.

ACKNOWLEDGEMENTS

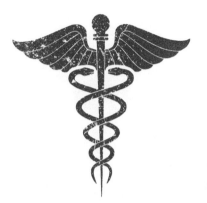

This is a book my patients and those individuals I interacted with during my lifetime helped to write.

As an author exploring the world of publishing, I benefited enormously from FreisenPress's generosity, encouragement, and the support staff who were always available when needed. The editors who edited my work were a blessing to the final product.

Finally, huge thanks to my late mom Mary Aziz Nakhla and big thanks to my best friend Margherita Greco and my friends in Europe in their encouragement and support.

ABOUT THE AUTHOR

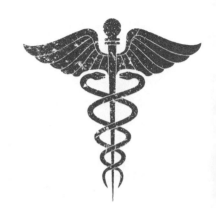

Nabil Basanti was born in Khartoum, Sudan, Africa in the year 1954. He lived there to the age of twenty-five, by which time he had completed all didactic courses and had graduated from the faculty of Medicine at the University of Khartoum which was affiliated with the Royal Colleges of Edinburgh and Dublin.

Dr. Basanti, after qualifying as a non-restricted practicing physician in Sudan and was registered with the Sudan Medical Council, started to explore specialization venues in the civilised world. He lived in America from 1982 to 1989 where he had his daughter and twin sons. The laws in the US at that time did not help him to achieve his goals. He returned to Sudan and practiced medicine as a general practitioner from 1989 to 1990.

Dr. Basanti had to flee Sudan for the safety of his family since there was discrimination against Christians and those having a fair complexion. He elected to have Canada as his home and was accepted as a conventional refugee according to the Geneva Convention. His medical qualifications were not accepted, though, and his MB.BS. Medical qualification was considered as a BSc in General Science from the University of Toronto. After passing the qualifying medical exams of the Canadian Medical Council, he was offered four different positions in different provinces, but the local boards refused to award him a temporary licence to practice. He elected to study Nuclear Medicine Technology to be able to obtain a certification to allow him to work as a technologist to bring up his three kids and provide for his family. In 1994, he graduated and was qualified as a Medical Radiation Technologist in Canada. He worked in Nuclear Medicine in different Canadian Hospitals and Independent Health facilities.

Dr. Basanti was previously the president, owner and director of GTA Nuclear Cardiology Ltd. an independent health facility from 2005 to 2007. He was a vice president and partner of Scarborough Nuclear Medicine Ltd from 2001 to 2003. In 2005, he obtained an MRI qualification from the British Colombia Institute of Technology with an honors degree. Contracted with a Regional hospital in Nova Scotia, Canada to modify, upgrade and implement protocols for their MRI department from 2008 to 2010. Dr. Basanti successfully controlled the MRI wait times and presented MRI wait time project solutions to different provincial ministries of health and the Canadian Military. None of the parties were interested to implement the solutions and elected to live with the wait time crisis.

Dr. Basanti was a professional member in the following:

> International Society for Magnetic Resonance in Medicine (ISMRM), USA

> American Registry of Radiological Technologists; RT. (MR) (ARRT), USA

About The Author

Canadian Association of Medical Radiation Technologists (CAMRT), Canada

College of Medical Radiation Technologists of Ontario (CMRTO), Canada

Canadian Society of Nuclear Medicine, Canada

Ontario Association of Medical Scientists (OAMS), Canada

Nuclear Medicine Technology Certification Board, USA

Australian and New Zealand Society of Nuclear Medicine, Australia

Society of Nuclear Medicine (Technologist Section), USA

Sudan Medical Council, Sudan

Dr. Basanti, from 2005 till present, is the president at Basanti Advisory Services which provides the following: advice, analysis, and recommendations for software/hardware development and upgrading of imaging sites' designs, setup and operations; PACS implementation; Review of existing protocols; Statistical analysis and report generation of utilization profiles; Recommendations for operational changes to increase efficiency and production; Create, design, implement, and follow up new innovative health projects to solve health system needs.

CPSIA information can be obtained
at www.ICGtesting.com
Printed in the USA
LVHW012240291119
638675LV00003B/124